T0259090

Professional Development for Psychiatrists

Editors

HOWARD Y. LIU
DONALD M. HILTY

PSYCHIATRIC CLINICS OF NORTH AMERICA

www.psych.theclinics.com

Consulting Editor
HARSH K. TRIVEDI

September 2019 • Volume 42 • Number 3

ELSEVIER

1600 John F. Kennedy Boulevard • Suite 1800 • Philadelphia, Pennsylvania, 19103-2899

http://www.theclinics.com

PSYCHIATRIC CLINICS OF NORTH AMERICA Volume 42, Number 3
September 2019 ISSN 0193-953X, ISBN-13: 978-0-323-66106-5

Editor: Lauren Boyle
Developmental Editor: Kristen Helm

Psychiatric Clinics of North America (ISSN 0193-953X) is published quarterly by Elsevier Inc., 360 Park Avenue South, New York, NY 10010-1710. Months of issue are March, June, September, and December. Business and Editorial Offices: 1600 John F. Kennedy Blvd., Suite 1800, Philadelphia, PA 19103-2899. Periodicals postage paid at New York, NY and additional mailing offices. Subscription prices are $332.00 per year (US individuals), $699.00 per year (US institutions), $100.00 per year (US students/residents), $406.00 per year (Canadian individuals), $462.00 per year (international individuals), $880.00 per year (Canadian & international institutions), and $220.00 per year (Canadian & international students/residents). Foreign air speed delivery is included in all *Clinics'* subscription prices. All prices are subject to change without notice. **POSTMASTER:** Send address changes to *Psychiatric Clinics of North America*, Elsevier Health Sciences Division, Subscription Customer Service, 3251 Riverport Lane, Maryland Heights, MO 63043. **Customer Service: 1-800-654-2452 (US). From outside the United States, call 1-314-447-8871. Fax: 1-314-447-8029. E-mail: journalscustomerservice-usa@elsevier.com (for print support) and journalsonline support-usa@elsevier.com (for online support).**

Reprints. For copies of 100 or more, of articles in this publication, please contact the Commercial Reprints Department, Elsevier Inc., 360 Park Avenue South, New York, New York 10010-1710. Tel.: 212-633-3874, Fax: 212-633-3820, E-mail: reprints@elsevier.com.

Psychiatric Clinics of North America is covered in *MEDLINE/PubMed (Index Medicus), Current Contents/Social and Behavioral Sciences, Social Science Citation Index, Embase/Excerpta Medica,* and PsycINFO.

Contributors

CONSULTING EDITOR

HARSH K. TRIVEDI, MD, MBA
President and Chief Executive Officer, Sheppard Pratt Health System, Baltimore, Maryland, USA

EDITORS

HOWARD Y. LIU, MD
Associate Professor and Chair, Department of Psychiatry, University of Nebraska Medical Center, Director, Behavioral Health Education Center of Nebraska, Omaha, Nebraska, USA

DONALD M. HILTY, MD, MBA
Associate Chief of Staff, Mental Health, VA Northern California Health Care System, Mather, California, USA; Professor and Vice-Chair, Department of Psychiatry and Behavioral Sciences, University of California, Davis, Davis, California, USA

AUTHORS

MARY S. AHN, MD
Vice Chair for Academic Affairs and Career Development, Director, Child and Adolescent Psychiatry Training, Associate Professor of Psychiatry and Pediatrics, Department of Psychiatry, University of Massachusetts Medical School, Worcester, Massachusetts, USA

SHADI AMINOLOLAMA-SHAKERI, MD
Associate Professor, Department of Radiology, University of California, Davis, Sacramento, California, USA

EUGENE V. BERESIN, MD, MA
Professor of Psychiatry, Harvard Medical School, Executive Director, The Clay Center for Young Healthy Minds, Massachusetts General Hospital, Boston, Massachusetts, USA

ROBERT J. BOLAND, MD
Vice Chair for Education, Department of Psychiatry, Brigham and Women's Hospital, Associate Professor, Harvard Medical School, Boston, Massachusetts, USA

JONATHAN BORUS, MD
Chairman Emeritus and Senior Psychiatrist, Brigham and Women's Hospital, Stanley Cobb Distinguished Professor of Psychiatry, Harvard Medical School, Boston, Massachusetts, USA

ELIZABETH BRANNAN, MD
Assistant Professor, Division of Child and Adolescent Psychiatry, The Warren Alpert Medical School of Brown University, Bradley Hospital, East Providence, Rhode Island, USA

STEVEN CHAN, MD, MBA
Physician, Addiction Treatment Services, VA Palo Alto Health Care System, University of California, San Francisco, Palo Alto, California, USA

MARGARET S. CHISOLM, MD
Professor of Psychiatry and Behavioral Sciences, Johns Hopkins Medicine, Baltimore, Maryland, USA

SANDRA M. DeJONG, MD, MSc
Assistant Professor, Department of Psychiatry, Cambridge Health Alliance, Harvard University School of Medicine, Cambridge Hospital, Cambridge, Massachusetts, USA

KENNETH P. DRUDE, PhD
Private Practice, Clinical Faculty Associate Professor, Wright State University, Fairborn, Ohio, USA

R. KEVIN GRIGSBY, MSW, DSW, ACSW
Senior Director, Member Organizational Development, Association of American Medical Colleges (AAMC), Washington, DC, USA

FREDERICK G. GUGGENHEIM, MD
Adjunct Professor of Psychiatry, University of Nebraska Medical Center College of Medicine, Omaha, Nebraska, USA; Professor of Psychiatry and Chair Emeritus, University of Arkansas for Medical Sciences, Little Rock, Arkansas, USA

DONALD M. HILTY, MD, MBA
Associate Chief of Staff, Mental Health, VA Northern California Health Care System, Mather, California, USA; Professor and Vice-Chair, Department of Psychiatry and Behavioral Sciences, University of California, Davis, Davis, California, USA

JEFFREY HUNT, MD
Professor and Program Director, Child and Adolescent Psychiatry Fellowship and Triple Board Program, Deputy Division Director, Division of Child and Adolescent Psychiatry, The Warren Alpert Medical School of Brown University, Bradley Hospital, East Providence, Rhode Island, USA

SHASHANK V. JOSHI, MD, FAAP, DFAACAP
Associate Professor of Psychiatry, Pediatrics, and Education, Director of Training in Child and Adolescent Psychiatry, Director of School Mental Health Services, Lucile Packard Children's Hospital at Stanford, Stanford, California, USA

RUTH LEVINE, MD
Clarence Ross Miller Professor, Department of Psychiatry and Behavioral Sciences, Associate Dean, Student Affairs and Admissions, School of Medicine, University of Texas Medical Branch, Galveston, Texas, USA

HOWARD Y. LIU, MD
Associate Professor and Chair, Department of Psychiatry, University of Nebraska Medical Center, Director, Behavioral Health Education Center of Nebraska, Omaha, Nebraska, USA

JOHN LUO, MD
Vice-Chair of Education and Program Director of Psychiatry Residency Training, University of California, Riverside, Department of Psychiatry, Riverside, California, USA

MARLENE MAHEU, PhD
Executive Director, Telebehavioral Health Institute, Inc., San Diego, California, USA

ALASTAIR J. S. McKEAN, MD
Assistant Professor, Department of Psychiatry and Psychology, Mayo Clinic, Rochester, Minnesota, USA

MYO THWIN MYINT, MD, FAAP, FAPA, DFAACAP
Assistant Professor of Psychiatry and Pediatrics, Department of Psychiatry and Behavioral Sciences, Program Director of Fellowship Training in Triple Board & Child and Adolescent Psychiatry Programs, Tulane University School of Medicine, New Orleans, Louisiana, USA

KEISUKE NAKAGAWA, MD
Postdoctoral Scholar, Department of Psychiatry and Behavioral Sciences, UC Davis Health, Sacramento, California, USA

ANDREEA L. SERITAN, MD
Professor, Department of Psychiatry, University of California, San Francisco, UCSF Weill Institute for Neurosciences, San Francisco, California, USA

SANDRA SEXSON, MD
Professor and Chief, Child, Adolescent and Family Psychiatry, Program Director, Child and Adolescent Psychiatry Residency Training, Department of Psychiatry and Health Behavior, Medical College of Georgia, Augusta University, Augusta, Georgia, USA

RUTH S. SHIM, MD, MPH
Luke and Grace Kim Professor in Cultural Psychiatry, Director of Cultural Psychiatry, Associate Professor, Department of Psychiatry and Behavioral Sciences, University of California, Davis, Sacramento, California, USA

ERICA Z. SHOEMAKER, MD, MPH
Chief of Clinical Services and Fellowship Program Director, Child and Adolescent Psychiatry, Clinical Associate Professor of Psychiatry and the Behavioral Sciences (Clinician Educator), Keck School of Medicine of USC, University of Southern California, LAC+ USC Medical Center, Los Angeles, California, USA

KARI A. SIMONSEN, MD
Assistant Vice Chancellor for Faculty Affairs, Vice Chair of Pediatrics, Chief, Pediatric Infectious Diseases, Professor of Pediatrics, University of Nebraska Medical Center, Omaha, Nebraska, USA

DOROTHY STUBBE, MD
Associate Professor, Child Study Center, Child and Adolescent Psychiatry, Program Director of Residency Training, Yale School of Medicine, New Haven, Connecticut, USA

JOHN TESHIMA, BSc, MEd, MD, FRCPC
Associate Professor, Department of Psychiatry, Sunnybrook Health Sciences Centre, University of Toronto, Toronto, Ontario, Canada

JOHN TOROUS, MD
Director, Digital Psychiatry Division, Department of Psychiatry, Beth Israel Deaconess Medical Center, Boston, Massachusetts, USA

JESSICA UNO, MD
Resident Physician, Psychiatry, Kaweah Delta Health Care District, Visalia, California, USA

JOEL YAGER, MD
Department of Psychiatry, University of Colorado School of Medicine, Aurora, Colorado, USA

PETER M. YELLOWLEES, MBBS, MD
Professor of Psychiatry, Department of Psychiatry and Behavioral Sciences, Chief Wellness Officer, UC Davis Health, Sacramento, California, USA

DOUGLAS ZIEDONIS, MD, MPH
Associate Vice Chancellor for Health Sciences, University of California, San Diego, Professor of Psychiatry, UC San Diego Health, La Jolla, California, USA

Contents

Professional development refers to training, formal education, and/or advanced professional learning intended to help clinicians, teachers, researchers, and administrators improve their professional knowledge and effectiveness. Institutions have been trying to adapt to a rapidly changing internal and external environment, with resource constraints and competitive health care. Professional development may be contextualized using adult development, educational, and organizational perspectives, and most best practices overlap. Key partners are faculty, departments, institutions, and national organizations. Interprofessional, team-based and project-based longitudinal initiatives may ignite educational innovations, and serve as a method to learn authentically in the workplace, promote socialization, and change attitudes.

Psychiatry's evolution has entailed clinical, educational, research, and administrative missions. Faculty development efforts concern ways in which professional identity, attitudes and skills are transmitted and enhanced from generation to generation. Top-down efforts by national and international organizations and bottom-up movements by individuals in numerous local settings have helped faculty and guided the profession forward. Organizations have provided new faculty with access to mentors and peers across the country, training opportunities, and up-to-date information on emerging scientific, pedagogical, and regulatory trends. Additional innovations and evaluation regarding best practices for faculty development initiatives in psychiatry are needed.

An academic career goes through developmental stages and faculty have different needs as they progress through these stages. Faculty development initiatives can target these developmental needs. Early career faculty develop their clinical and academic identities and benefit from orientation programs and mentorship. Mid-career faculty engage in role transitions, consolidating their careers, and focusing on productivity and generativity.

They benefit from programs that provide new skills, including leadership skills. Advanced career faculty focus on professional-personal integration, contributing to a community, and changes in roles and power. They can benefit from mentorship, from peers locally and at a distance.

Clinical faculty need creative, systematic, and supportive approaches for their success. Academic institutions and departments have a unique opportunity to engage its faculty by sponsoring and creating innovative professional development programs to enhance leadership, research, teaching, and clinical skills. The added benefit of these "homegrown" programs is that clinical faculty members feel more valued, engaged, and supported and will want to better align their priorities with the strategic priorities of the institution. There are excellent national resources to learn from to support and complement local professional development efforts. Each department needs to balance any standard with customized approaches.

Ongoing professional development is essential across the career development life span. Coaching is emerging as an effective intervention to support career, personal, and leadership development of both individuals and teams in health care, given the high levels of volatility, uncertainty, complexity, and ambiguity that our physicians and organizations face. Coaches, in contrast to mentors, avoid giving direct advice to clients, while still providing self-awareness and other-awareness and accountability to their goals. The use of coaches increases the flexibility of supporting our psychiatrists with a team of supporters, distilling the time of busy mentors to advise primarily on their content expertise.

Projects done in interprofessional groups can foster faculty development with minimal resources beyond what is already available at the university or medical center. Each project can yield multiple "wins" in individual faculty growth while meeting the needs of academic medical centers. These projects can build collaborative skills and a sense of community among faculty, trainees, and staff. The combination of low costs, high yields, and improvements in team skills make these approaches appealing and sustainable in resource-constrained medical centers. The authors describe 4 sample projects and their teams, needed resources, and outcomes.

The American Board of Medical Specialties, which includes the American Board of Psychiatry and Neurology, promotes standards focusing on changes in physicians' medical knowledge and skills. The authors describe the literature concerning the effectiveness of lifelong learning. They review the status of the American Board of Psychiatry and Neurology Maintenance of Certification program as an example of a model of lifelong learning, including an innovative pilot. The final sections include a discussion of new innovations to consider in continuing professional development and a reflection about the state of lifelong learning within the context of maintenance of certification in psychiatry.

R. Kevin Grigsby

Many leaders consider engaging in formal leadership training that results in the award of a degree. Choosing from several options requires careful consideration given the cost, effort, and attention required for successful completion. Individuals should have a clear understanding as to motivation for pursuing an advanced degree and should be able to clearly articulate what they hope to gain. If the motivation is driven by desire for yet another credential, one is ill advised to enroll in a program. Graduate degrees in business, health administration, public administration, public health, medical management, and organizational leadership are described, and learning format options.

Kenneth P. Drude, Marlene Maheu, and Donald M. Hilty

In the ever-changing fields of health care, continuing professional development (CPD) and lifelong learning are essential for patient care, regulatory requirements, personal growth, and job satisfaction. However, no specific systems in approaching CPD have been delineated, and most health professionals are left to their own devices to manage it, on top of all their other professional responsibilities. This article (1) outlines the importance of CPD, (2) describes potential systematic approaches to CPD and potential ways to assess their effectiveness, and (3) reviews resources available to incorporate into a systematic approach.

Kari A. Simonsen and Ruth S. Shim

Recognizing and embracing culture, diversity, and inclusion is essential to the practice of high-quality clinical care in medicine and, more specifically, in psychiatry. When leadership lacks diversity, the organizational policies and norms may skew toward devaluing the importance of diversity and inclusion. Considering the significant underrepresentation at the academic faculty level, substantive individual and systemic efforts are required to recruit, retain, and advance a diverse and inclusive student pipeline and faculty in academic psychiatry. For meaningful progress to be made, leaders in psychiatry must resemble an increasingly diverse field of psychiatry residents who serve a more diverse community of patients.

dimensions like clinical decision support, technology selection, and information flow management across an e-platform. Health systems must integrate in-person and technology-based care, while maintaining the therapeutic relationship.

Editorial

Frederick G. Guggenheim

> Navigating and negotiating the stages from instructor to assistant, associate, and full professor to chair is an exciting, if at times exhausting, journey. Becoming a member of an academic department has the allure, and burden, of participating in, and supporting a community of scholars. In addition to proceeding through their career considerations, faculty members go through their own adult developmental stages. Suggested issues to consider that may enhance faculty members' opportunities in academia are listed. The tenure rules and the culture of each department, plus the priorities of the chair, become important when choosing to invest in a new department.

Professional Development for Psychiatrists

PSYCHIATRIC CLINICS OF NORTH AMERICA

FORTHCOMING ISSUES

December 2019
Integrating Technology into 21st Century Psychiatry: Telemedicine, Social Media, and other Technologies
James H. Shore, *Editor*

March 2020
Mixed Affective States: Beyond Current Boundaries
Alan C. Swann and Gabriele Sani, *Editors*

RECENT ISSUES

June 2019
Eating Disorders: Part II
Harry A. Brandt and Steven F. Crawford, *Editors*

March 2019
Eating Disorders: Part I
Harry A. Brandt and Steven F. Crawford, *Editors*

SERIES OF RELATED INTEREST

Child and Adolescent Psychiatric Clinics of North America
Neurologic Clinics

Preface

The Central Role of Professional Development and Psychiatry

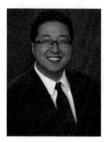 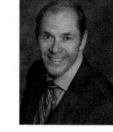

Howard Y. Liu, MD   Donald M. Hilty, MD, MBA
Editors

The pace of new knowledge and new skills is ever accelerating in health care. Professional development (PD) is necessary to equip physicians and other health care providers with the skills to adapt to new roles, respond to challenges, and integrate new knowledge into their clinical practices. In this issue, Hilty and colleagues have defined PD as a wide variety of specialized training, formal education, and/or advanced professional learning intended to help clinicians, teachers, researchers, and administrators improve their professional knowledge, competence, skill, and effectiveness. It encompasses continuing medical education, faculty development, and other forms of lifelong learning.

Several trends in health care have converged to challenge existing paradigms in PD, requiring a more nuanced survey of the field. First, faculty development and faculty affairs offices have emerged in academic health centers, creating centralized resources to foster mentoring, educational skills development, and career guidance to academic physicians.[1] This has led to a greater sophistication of efforts to accelerate faculty skills development in clinical, educational, research, and administrative domains. Second, technology continues to innovate and disrupt all aspects of health care, with health systems prioritizing continuing PD and continuing medical education to improve service delivery, quality, and efficiency.[2,3] Technology is being used to organize, integrate, and evaluate practice systems, and e-portfolios and social media are used similarly, to network, track learning outcomes, and facilitate teamwork across distance. Third, as health care disparities continue to impact population health, there is a growing recognition that we must foster a diverse psychiatry workforce to provide culturally and

Psychiatr Clin N Am 42 (2019) xiii–xv
https://doi.org/10.1016/j.psc.2019.05.015
0193-953X/19/© 2019 Published by Elsevier Inc.

linguistically appropriate care to all patients and all communities.[4] The PD needs of women and underrepresented minorities must be explicitly addressed to cultivate the future leaders we need. Finally, increasing complexities of the health care economy have challenged the ability of physicians to navigate an ever-shifting regulatory and payer system.

This issue was organized to address the new realities of PD in psychiatry in the twenty-first century. Authors include past and present chairs of psychiatry, an associate vice chancellor of research, an interim assistant vice chancellor for faculty affairs, acclaimed program directors, national leaders in lifelong learning, vice chairs of education, a certified executive coach, and the Senior Director of Member Organizational Development at the Association of American Medical Colleges. It also includes physicians at various stages of career from a resident physician to a retired professor emeritus. This issue pairs women physicians with expertise in faculty development and cultural psychiatry in highlighting the importance of diversity and inclusion in psychiatric leadership. The issue is organized into the following 4 themes:

1. The landscape of PD;
2. A discussion of approaches to PD;
3. A review of diversity, wellness, and transitions; and
4. A review of technology and its increasing role in PD.

The editors are appreciative of their own mentors in the field of faculty development. Dr Liu would like to thank 3 amazing women faculty mentors who taught him the principles and the responsibility of those who lead PD to shape the future of the profession: Dr Luanne Thorndyke, Dr Myrna Newland, and Dr Linda M. Love. Dr Hilty would like to thank many mentors, colleagues, and mentees: Dr Robert E. Hales; Dr Joel Yager; fellows, residents, and medical students; and most importantly, early career faculty, who have collaborated and shared ideas, ups and downs, and time in helping patients and learners of all walks of life.

In the words of Supreme Court Justice, Ruth Bader Ginsburg, "Real change, enduring change, happens one step at a time." At its core, PD fosters continuous calibration of skills to the challenges we face in psychiatry and medicine. This process is contextualized using adult development, education, and organizational perspectives. It is also based on systematic assessment of needs and best practices, which provide both structure and organized processes for faculty, departments, institutions, and organizations to be successful.

ACKNOWLEDGMENTS

The editors would like to acknowledge the following individuals: Robert E. Hales, MD, MBA, Emeritus Joe P. Tupin Professor and Chair, Department of Psychiatry and Behavioral Sciences, University of California, Davis School of Medicine, Sacramento, CA. Linda M. Love, EdD, Director of Faculty Development Programs, University of Nebraska Medical Center, Omaha, NE. Myrna Newland, MD, Former Director of Faculty Development Programs and Professor Emeritus of Anesthesiology, University of Nebraska Medical Center, Omaha, NE. Luanne Thorndyke, MD, Vice Provost for Faculty Affairs and Professor of Medicine, University of Massachusetts Medical School, Waltham, MA. H. Dele Davies, MD, Senior Vice Chancellor for Academic

Affairs, University of Nebraska Medical Center, Omaha, NE. Joel Yager, MD, Professor, Department of Psychiatry, University of Colorado School of Medicine, Aurora, CO.

Howard Y. Liu, MD
Department of Psychiatry
University of Nebraska Medical Center
985575 Nebraska Medical Center
Omaha, NE, 68198-5575, USA

Donald M. Hilty, MD, MBA
Northern California Veterans Administration
Health Care System
Department of Psychiatry and
Behavioral Sciences
10535 Hospital Way
Mather, CA 95655, USA

University of California Davis
Sacramento, CA 95817, USA

E-mail addresses:
hyliu@unmc.edu (H.Y. Liu)
donh032612@gmail.com (D.M. Hilty)

REFERENCES

1. Sonnino RE, Reznik V, Thorndyke LA, et al. Evolution of faculty affairs and faculty development offices in US Medical Schools: a 10-year follow-up survey. Acad Med 2013;88:1368–75.
2. Wallace S, May SA. Assessing and enhancing quality through outcomes-based continuing professional development (CPD): a review of current practice. Vet Rec 2016;179(20):515–20.
3. Opperman C, Liebig D, Bowling J, et al. Measuring return on investment for professional development activities: 2018 Updates. J Nurses Prof Dev 2018;34(6):303–12.
4. Nivet MA. A diversity 3.0 update: are we moving the needle enough? Acad Med 2015;90(12):1591–3.

Defining Professional Development in Medicine, Psychiatry, and Allied Fields

Donald M. Hilty, MD, MBA[a],*, Howard Y. Liu, MD[b,c],
Dorothy Stubbe, MD[d], John Teshima, BSc, MEd, MD, FRCPC[e]

KEYWORDS

- Professional • Development • Medicine • Psychiatry • Faculty • Organization
- Profession • Career

KEY POINTS

- Professional development is training, formal education, and/or advanced professional learning intended to help faculty improve their professional knowledge, skills, and effectiveness.
- Professional development may be contextualized using adult development, education, and organizational perspectives.
- Systematic assessment of needs and best practices provides both structure and organized processes for departments, institutions, and organizations.
- Initiatives in professional development for women, underrepresented minorities, and other populations are improving, but further progress is needed.

INTRODUCTION

Professional development (PD) refers to a wide variety of specialized training, formal education, and/or advanced professional learning intended to help clinicians, teachers, researchers, and administrators improve their professional knowledge, competence, skill, and effectiveness. Faculty, departments, and institutions have been trying to address PD challenges in a rapidly changing, resource-constrained, and

Disclosure: The authors have nothing to disclose.
[a] Mental Health, Northern California Veterans Administration Health Care System, Department of Psychiatry and Behavioral Sciences, University of California Davis, 10535 Hospital Way, Mather, Sacramento, CA 95655, USA; [b] Department of Psychiatry, University of Nebraska Medical Center, 42nd and Emile, Omaha, NE 68198, USA; [c] Behavioral Health Education Center of Nebraska, Omaha, NE, USA; [d] Child Study Center, Child and Adolescent Psychiatry, Yale School of Medicine, 230 South Frontage Road, New Haven, CT 06519, USA; [e] Department of Psychiatry, Sunnybrook Health Sciences Centre, University of Toronto, 2075 Bayview Avenue, Room FG-62, Toronto, Ontario M4N 3M5, Canada
* Corresponding author. VA Northern California Health Care System, 10535 Hospital Way, Mather, CA 95655, USA.
E-mail address: donh032612@gmail.com

Psychiatr Clin N Am 42 (2019) 337–356
https://doi.org/10.1016/j.psc.2019.04.001
0193-953X/19/Crown Copyright © 2019 Published by Elsevier Inc. All rights reserved.

competitive environment.[1] For example, departments and institutions (eg, academic health centers [AHCs]) must adapt to internal and external forces that change technology, operational processes, and administrative requirements. Health systems have prioritized continuing PD (CPD) and continuing medical education (CME) for service delivery to improve the quality, timeliness, and efficiency of systems,[2,3] and partly because of concerns about cost and return on investment.[4,5] Overall, CME has more of a positive impact on physician performance than patient health outcomes.[6]

Faculty development (FD) refers to the enhancement and reinforcement of academic roles, which include education, leadership, and research. The mission of FD requires definition, programming, funding, and a culture for success. FD generally also refers to that broad range of activities that institutions use to assist faculty in balancing, integrating, and changing their multiple roles.[7,8] PD may also include entrepreneurial, consulting, and leadership roles related to organizational change.[9] Education/training, clinical care, leadership, and PD or FD missions are valued, but less well organized, assessed, and funded than research. PD related to leadership is also increasing.[10] All areas require alignment between outcomes and evaluation, and progress is substantially related to effectiveness and translational efforts. Even more basic to this evolution is that the design, implementation, and evaluation of FD activities be informed by the most up-to-date research: the concept of knowledge translation (KT).[11]

Without adequate FD, faculty attrition increases and the cost of faculty replacement is staggering in financial (eg, a single generalist and specialist at \$115,554 and \$286,503, respectively) and nonfinancial terms.[12] Even when rigorous FD interventions show gains in knowledge, skills, and teaching behavior changes, such as enhanced teaching practices, new educational initiatives, new leadership positions, and increased academic output, permanent organizational changes to facilitate FD are infrequently explored.[13] The American Association of Medical Colleges (AAMC) Group on Faculty Affairs has increasingly evaluated these issues as part of its effort to build and sustain faculty vitality in medical schools and teaching hospitals, as well as helping faculty affairs deans and administrators with institutional policies and PD activities.

Medicine and the health professions have collaborated in many circles, perhaps most influentially within the AAMC,[14] the Professional and Organizational Development (POD) Higher Education Network,[15] and the Association for Medical Education in Europe (AMEE). Historically, representatives of 22 medical schools met in Philadelphia in 1876 and formed the provisional AAMC to consider reform of medical college work.[14] The organization focuses on equitable health care; research; system sustainability; and a culturally competent, diverse workforce. POD's mission since 1976 has been to advance the research and practice of educational development in higher education. It has international conferences for networking, best practices, and producing publications, including the Guide to Faculty Development.[15] The interface of organizational development and business (eg, the 4Ps of product, price, place, and promotion) is notable with the POD Network. AMEE currently promotes best practices and scholarship in FD.[16]

The evolution of psychiatry is interwoven with those of medicine and science, providing context on how the field's identity has changed over time (**Table 1**). The American Psychiatric Association (APA) was founded in 1844 and the American Medical Association (AMA) in 1847. Psychiatry has had fundamental shifts by integrating opposites: narrative with descriptive, subjective with objective, and artistic and mysterious with scientific.[17] From the eighteenth century to the current era of patient-centered care, the field has helped society begin to address orphan medical topics and reduce stigma related to mental illness (eg, Pinel unchaining psychiatric and neurologic patients in the nineteenth century).[17] Although the National Institutes of Health was established in 1887, the National Institute of Mental Health (NIMH) only became a separate entity in 1947.

Table 1
Key historical developments in psychiatry and medicine that provide context for professional development

Time Period	Event
1600s–1800s	
1656	Pitié-Salpêtrière Hospital in Paris opens
1783	Bicêtre Hospital, Paris, for the "mentally defective," chains removed from patients
1808	German physician Johann Christian Reil used the term psychiatry
1812	Benjamin Rush advocates for humane treatment of the mentally ill in *Medical Inquiries and Observations Upon Diseases of the Mind*, the first American textbook on psychiatry
1844	American Psychiatric Association founded
1847	American Medical Association founded
1876	Association of American Medical Colleges founded
1887	National Institutes of Health founded
1893	German psychiatrist Emil Kraepelin clinically defined dementia praecox, later reformulated as schizophrenia
1895	Sigmund Freud and Josef Breuer, Austria, *Studies on Hysteria*
1895	"How soon can a child go mad?" by Harold Maudsley, in *The Pathology of the Mind*
1900s	
1900–1930s	Classical conditioning (Pavlov), operant conditioning (Skinner)
1902	Adolf Meyer became director of the New York State Psychiatric Institute: medical model, records and "common sense"
1905	Binet-Simon Test, the first intelligence test
1908	Paul Eugene Bleuler, Switzerland, Uses the term schizophrenia
1911	American Psychoanalytic Association founded
1913	Carl Jung, analytical psychology
1917	Object relations theory, with Ferenczi and later British psychologists Melanie Klein, Donald Winnicott, 1940s and 1950s
1920	Hermann Rorschach developed the Rorschach Inkblot Test
1927	Julius Wagner-Jauregg, Austrian psychiatrist, Nobel Prize in Physiology or Medicine, 1927, therapeutic value of malaria inoculation in the treatment of dementia paralytica
1927	Manfred Sakel, Austrian psychiatrist, insulin shock therapy as a treatment of psychosis; discontinued in 1970s
1932	Jean Piaget, cognitive theory, publication of his work *The Moral Judgment of Children*
1934	The American Board of Psychiatry and Neurology, Inc. founded
1938	Italian neurologist Ugo Cerletti and Italian psychiatrist Dr Lucio Bini discovered electroconvulsive therapy
1942	American Psychosomatic Society founded Carl Rogers, client-centered therapy
1946	National Mental Health Act, funding for National Institute of Mental Health, out of concern for public and veterans
1947	Antonio Egas Moniz, Nobel Prize, 1949, for his discovery of the therapeutic value of leucotomy in certain psychoses

(continued on next page)

Table 1 *(continued)*	
Time Period	**Event**
1948	Lithium carbonate's ability to stabilize mood demonstrated by Australian psychiatrist John Cade, first effective medicine for the treatment of mental illness
1949	NIMH established and funding for children in 1970s
1950	The World Psychiatric Association founded
1952	APA published the first DSM; revised in 1968, 1980/1987, 1994, 2000, and 2013
1953	American Academy of Child and Adolescent Psychiatry founded Academy for Consultation-Liaison Psychiatry (formerly Academy of Psychosomatic Medicine) founded
1954	Abraham Maslow, *Motivation and Personality* and hierarchy of needs
1950s-1970s	First monoamine oxidase inhibitor, antipsychotic, and benzodiazepine developed Developmental psychology flourished after World War I with Jean Piaget (Switzerland), Lev Vygotsky (Russia), and John Bowlby (United Kingdom) Telepsychiatry (video) launches
1960s	Aaron T. Beck developed cognitive therapy
1963	Community Mental Health Centers Act
1956	NIMH founded the Career Teachers Program
1967	NIMH began independent of the National Institutes of Health
1970	American Association of Directors of Psychiatric Residency Training founded
1970	Society for Academic Psychiatry founded; became Association for Academic Psychiatry in 1971
1974	Association of Directors of Medical Student Education in Psychiatry founded
1977	Biopsychosocial model was proposed by George L. Engel
1977	President Jimmy Carter's Presidential Commission on Mental Health
1977	The International Classification of Diseases-9 was published by the World Health Organization
1980s	Handheld phone introduced
1981	National Alliance for Research on Schizophrenia and Depression
1990	Mental Health America advocates for Americans with Disabilities Act
1990s	Modern telemedicine and telepsychiatry launches
1994	The Mental Health Parity Act by President Clinton APA Outline for Cultural Formulation in DSM-IV
1996	The International Classification of Diseases-10 was published by the World Health Organization
2000s	
2000	Eric R. Kandel, Nobel Prize in Physiology or Medicine, for discoveries concerning signal transduction in the nervous system
2000	Genetic researchers map human genes with the aim of isolating the individual chromosome responsible for mental dysfunction
2003	President's (Clinton) New Freedom Commission on Mental Health, *Achieving the Promise: Transforming Mental Health Care in America*
2008	Mental Health Parity Act

(continued on next page)

Table 1 (continued)	
Time Period	**Event**
2010	The Patient Protection and Affordable Care Act (P.L. 111–148), (health care reform law signed by President Obama)
2012	Brian K. Kobilka, Stanford University, Nobel Prize in Chemistry, 2012, the communication system between G-protein–coupled receptors and body
2013	DSM-5
2014	John O'Keefe, May-Britt Moser, and Edvard Moser, Nobel Prize, cells that constitute a positioning system in the brain key to memory

Abbreviations: APA, American Psychiatric Association; DSM, diagnostic and statistical manual of mental disorders; NIMH, National Institute of Mental Health.

The profession of psychiatry and its FD path was forged through many key events in the twentieth century. Help to individuals with trauma after World War II solidified the role of psychiatry and psychotherapy, because healing by listening to patient stories was seen as instrumental. Exploration of the medicine-psychiatry interface led to the Academy of Psychosomatic Medicine in 1953 (now Academy for Consultation-Liaison Psychiatry), and the biopsychosocial model modestly organized clinical assessment and treatment.[18] Modern descriptive psychiatry began in 1968, building on what Kraepelin and others put forward. The academic organizations arrived in the 1970s with footing from the NIMH (eg, American Association of Directors of Psychiatric Residency Training [AADPRT], 1970; Association for Academic Psychiatry [AAP], 1971, initially called the Society for Academic Psychiatry; Association of Directors of Medical Student Education in Psychiatry [ADMSEP], 1975).

This article discusses PD; specifically:

1. Why it is relevant, how it is defined, and its intersection with adult development and education
2. Its core outcomes/targets and the structures and processes used by faculty, departments, and institutions to achieve PD
3. How it is evolving to promote innovations in educational methods, which may be more systematically approached and studied

The literature covered is tilted toward the US evolution, but with international contributions on best practices and innovations. Several related areas are not discussed (eg, academic personnel/administration, responsible for supervision, educational policy, and academic programs; faculty affairs, which may have joint responsibilities with PD). Other articles in this special edition speak at length to topics raised here, including CPD related to lifelong learning and faculty needs within specific career stages; a particular challenge is defining, assessing, and programming related to mid-career faculty, which have to juggle academic scholarship, service, and leadership endeavors.[19] Other topics of importance are covered elsewhere (eg, PD for adjunct and part-time faculty) and within the international literature on PD.

PROFESSIONAL AND/OR FACULTY DEVELOPMENT: CORE COMPONENTS AND PERSPECTIVES ON CONTEXT

The initial push for PD or FD came as a result of faculty being ill-prepared to teach in graduate and health profession education,[20] which led to instructional units at undergraduate institutions, which focused on teaching skills, evaluation, and other topics.[21]

The first support for FD may have been a sabbatical at Harvard University in 1810.[22] In undergraduate circles, the historical evolution in FD includes eras over time: Age of the Scholar, Age of the Teacher, Age of the Developer, Age of the Learner, and now Age of the Network.[22] The goal of this age is to preserve, clarify, and enhance the purposes of FD, and to network with faculty and institutional leaders.

In medical education, review articles have mapped out the scope and many approaches to PD or FD.[23,24] FD spans clinical, educational, research, and administrative activities[13,25]; others included leadership and management[9,10,26] (**Table 2**). Typically, the goal is to improve faculty knowledge and skills in the areas of teaching, research, administration,[27] and training for students and residents.[28] Institutions have traditionally focused on mentoring for academic productivity in medicine, as well as highly structured and well-mentored MD/PhD and early career award programs for research.[29]

An understanding of PD in academic medicine requires definitions and context. Faculty is usually defined in health systems as all individuals who are involved in the teaching and education of learners at all levels of the education continuum (eg, undergraduate, graduate, postgraduate, continuing); leadership and management in the university, the hospital, and the community; and research and scholarship, across the health professions (eg, social sciences, nursing, informatics). The terms, scope, and emphases differ across cultures and languages. The context for PD relates to the expectation of excellence in science and health care, both in providing outstanding care and training future generations. for the goal is a culture of academic vitality, manifest by alignment of personal and professional values within the organization.[30] The Royal College of Physicians and Surgeons of Canada maintenance of certification program recognizes FD as a critical element in maintaining professional standards.[31]

PD has been performed through teaching and learning through a variety of models that parallel adult education.[32] For the greatest part of its history, the predominate model of PD has been the apprenticeship model, which assumes that learning is facilitated when people work on authentic tasks in real settings of application or practice. This model serves as the foundation for other cognitive structures and the development of skilled competence.[32,33] With this comes a transformation of the learners' identity as they adopt the language, values, and practices of a specific social group. The developmental perspective/model, founded on the constructivist orientation to learning, aims to develop increasingly complex and sophisticated ways of reasoning and problem solving within a content area or field of practice. This model is based on sociologic, educational, and psychological research, which shows that learning may be enhanced by aligning teaching methods with learner attributes and goals, resulting in cognitive knowledge, attitudes, or skills acquisition. For systems and institutions, combining the apprenticeship and developmental perspectives may work, similar to the way clinicians are reacculturated into new communities of practices and ways of thinking.[34]

Another way to frame PD is theory of the process of teacher change.[35] There are 6 interrelated perspectives on how teachers change, all of which could apply to the PD in the health professions:

1. Training: change is something that is done to teachers
2. Adaptation: teachers change (or adapt) in response to changed condition
3. Personal development: teachers seek to change in an attempt to improve performance or develop new skills
4. Local reform: teachers change something for reasons of personal growth

Table 2
How departments, institutions, and national organizations help meet professional development needs

Area of Need	Department	Institution/Health System	International/National Professional Organizations
Clinical			
Knowledge	Subject matter expertise basic and specialized areas of interest	Customized application of psychiatric expertise to medical settings	Board certification and recertification, including subspecialty, if applicable
Skill	Provide basic and specialized care in area of interest in psychiatry; supervision; role modeling	Adapt assessment, triage, and management skills to population/setting; apply data to practice	Improvement in practice for psychiatry and subspecialty, if applicable
Team	Promote attitudes, communication, and efficiency at top of license	Engage across departments, services, and systems; ethics; professionalism	Interface of micro (eg, team, service) and macro (system) issues
Interprofessional education	Promote collaborative learning and quality of care between mental health disciplines	Share mental models and collaborate between psychiatry and medicine	System issues across schools, professions, and institutions
Education/Teaching			
Knowledge	Content and process; identify outcomes	Evaluation, intervention, and research; competency and expertise concepts	Specialized, collaborative experiences with peers and mentors
Learner-centeredness	Engagement; customized assessment; incremental plan; positive climate	Exposure to broader concepts (eg, content, learner, and teacher triad)	Consultation, in-depth evaluation, qualitative and quantitative
Interpersonal and communication skill	Communicate expectations; provide feedback; encourage reflection	Adapt to additional peers/disciplines and learner levels; use feedback	Social and difficult situation analysis for reassessment and intervention
Methodology and planning	Assess learners, setting; align outcomes and methods	Adapt methods (eg, problem, case, and team based)	System and resource issues; integration of clinical and education missions

(continued on next page)

Table 2
(continued)

Area of Need	Department	Institution/Health System	International/National Professional Organizations
Research/Scholarship			
Attitude of inquiry	Peers, mentor; journal clubs, grand rounds; need for data; reflection	Data options and processes; quality improvement; intramural resources	International/national expectations, experience, and perspective
Design and methodology	Mentor, peer, and team activities; cross-sectional/short-term course	Intramural, state/regional vs extramural; biostatistical services	Federal grant panels, funding organizations
Evaluation	Peer review, works in progress,	Consultation on specialized (eg, cost) and interdisciplinary areas	New directions and methods; changing metrics and paradigms
Writing, scholarship, and dissemination	Seminars for internal peer review; case, chapter and article options	Didactics, longitudinal seminars, and workgroups for best practices	Best practices, guidelines, and special editions; editor/editorial boards
Administration			
Clinical care	Team leader; service and/or medical director	Institutional, state, and regional practices and requirements	Federal (eg, Joint Commission, Centers for Medicare & Medicaid Services)
Leadership	Committee, course, or program director	Course or committee leader; director or other dean's office position	Representative, officer, president of organization; board member/leader
Budget, finance	Service, site (ie, clinical) and/or study (eg, research) prioritization	Interface of finance/reimbursement with resource allocation	Executive training (eg, masters in business administration)
People and resources	Credentialing/peer review; management of team, hospital	Human resources, academic affairs/personnel; quality improvement	Executive training (eg, Six Sigma, Lean)

5. Systemic restructuring: teachers enact the change policies of the system
6. Growth or learning: teachers change through professional activity

The current view of FD activities in the health professions seems to align primarily with the notion of change as training and personal development.[9]

PD has been contextualized related to successful aging and its 6 domains (or perspectives).[36] These are:

1. Physician-assessed objective physical health (and the absence of irreversible physical disability)
2. Subjective physical health
3. Longitudinal active life
4. Objective mental health, which refers to work, relationships, play, and the absence of need for psychiatric care or medication
5. Subjective life satisfaction related to marriage, job, children, and friendship
6. Social supports (eg, friends, spouse, and children)

The larger frame of reference is fundamentally Erikson's[37] (1963) model, to which Vaillant[36] added additional stages. After Erikson's[37] identity versus identity confusion stage, Vaillant[36] added career consolidation, in which adults find a job that is valuable to society and to themselves. Four developmental criteria seem to transform a job or hobby into a career: contentment, compensation, competence, and commitment. Erikson's[37] generativity, in which people manifest care for the next generation in a broad social sense, is key to mentoring and FD, as people unselfishly guide the next generation and give of themselves. This criterion may be manifest in community building as a consultant, guide, mentor, or coach to young adults in the larger society. Vaillant[36] added another dimension to this, called keeper of the meaning, which involves passing on the traditions of the past to the next generation.[36] People should see all sides (or not take sides) on an issue, and the focus is on the building and preservation of collective products and the culture in which people live and of its institutions.

THE EVOLUTION OF PROFESSIONAL DEVELOPMENT IN PSYCHIATRY: KEY FEATURES AND CONTRIBUTING PARTNERS

In the 1960s, the NIMH funded paths in psychiatry, residency education, and family medicine that highlighted knowledge and skills related to mental health and/or retraining in psychiatry. This process set the stage for academic organizations that arrived in the 1970s: AADPRT, 1970; Association For Academic Psychiatry, 1971; ADMSEP, 1975. Modern descriptive psychiatry began in 1968 and most recently produced the Diagnostic and Statistical Manual of Mental Disorders, Fifth Edition (DSM-5), 2013.[38] Genetic researchers mapped human genes with the aim of isolating the individual chromosome responsible for mental dysfunction in 2000. Presidential mental health commissions (1977, 2003) and the Mental Health Parity Act (2008) have also been formative.[26] Clinicians face new challenges from patient-centered care, evolving diseases, information "explosion," and emerging technologies.

Mentoring is a hallmark of FD programs and departments, and it includes preparation, training, and support. It also should be based on setting outcomes for academic productivity and/or career development more broadly (eg, socialization, satisfaction, self-efficacy).[39] The transmission perspective is probably the most common orientation to teaching in secondary and higher education, although not in adult education. Herein, effective teaching starts with a substantial commitment and mastery of the content or subject matter. Teachers must provide clear objectives, be organized and systematic, begin with fundamentals and adjust over time, clarify misunderstandings/answer questions, and provide feedback in order to reach high standards for achievement. Overall, good mentoring starts with assessment of faculty needs rather than departmental and organizational priorities.[22]

The concept of KT is fundamental to FD in many ways,[11] with origins in public health, medicine, and rehabilitation research.[40–42] KT is a term used to describe a process designed to address a long-standing issue: the underuse of available scientific findings and evidence-based research in systems of care.[41] KT is considered an interactive, nonlinear, and interdisciplinary process used to move knowledge into practice and includes all the steps between the creation of new knowledge and its application.[11] A direct link between KT and FD programs is simple: the best knowledge and scientific evidence is translated into methods for best practices, regardless of which paradigm (eg, positivism, postpositivism, interpretivism, and critical theory) for medical education research is used.[43]

Another major movement in PD, as is the case for clinical care, is the role of technology. Research suggests it can serve as a catalyst for the changes in the content, roles, and organizational climate and that a shift from traditional to constructivist instructional practices is needed.[44] The integration of US Department of Education's Office of Educational Technology Plan[45] with business (eg, IBM)[46] and learning theory[47] suggests that technology may transform, not just facilitate, teaching and organizational practices.[44] For CPD, competencies became available for telepsychiatry in 2015, telebehavioral health in 2017, and social media and mobile health/apps (2018).[48–52] Technology facilitates real-time patient and collegial interaction (eg, personal and professional Web sites to access information about health, doctors/faculty, departments, and AHCs) and dissemination scholarship (eg, via blogs, tweets, chats, and other options). Technology (eg, teleconferencing) has been used for mentoring, research, and education across geography (eg, University of Toronto Centre for Faculty Development).[44]

Institutional factors may facilitate and/or impede PD. Not all institutions have requisite technological, operational process, and administrative infrastructure related to health care resource constraints.[1] The context in which faculty members work, in which the institutional norms and policies reward and regulate their behavior, clearly influence their professional growth.[53] For example, some health profession schools and organizations provide PD opportunities and encourage experimentation with new ideas. Others may discourage such behaviors and may not lend administrative support to innovation and scholarship. In addition to competencies at the mentor level, institutional competences for teaching[54] and clinical care (eg, telepsychiatry)[48] have been suggested, with several domains: patient-centered care; measurable outcomes; trainee/student needs/roles; faculty clinical, teaching, and leadership roles/skills; institutional culture and process; finance, organizational structure, and funding; change management; and AHC-community partnerships.

A pivotal issue is how the profession passes on identity, attitudes, and skills to current and future generations.[55] Faculty have had to take initiative, collaborate with others, and seize opportunities because of diffusion of responsibility among departments and institutions, but academic organizations are playing a key role in PD in psychiatry. Because there are few directors/vice-chairs in departments and FD is dispersed between many associate/executive deans, there remains a diffusion of responsibility for who should do what among the many participants. In psychiatry, historically, academic organizations have propelled FD directly (eg, AAP), via training missions (eg, AADPRT, ADMSEP), and with master educator series[56] and surveys of needs.[57] Faculty share expertise and collaborate on projects and learning in many tangible/intangible ways.[58,59] Chairs and other stewards also need faculty and leadership development,[60] particularly those whose efforts focus almost exclusively on research. Because a standard academic approach for FD is lacking, the Accreditation Council of Graduate Medical Education has increasingly added requirements.

BEST PRACTICES FROM FIELDS/DISCIPLINES/PROFESSIONS IN/OUT OF MEDICINE

Some faculty are successful seeking mentoring (ie, antennae), whereas others need structure and organized processes from departments, institutions, and organizations. Therefore, systematic assessment of needs is suggested.[61] Although the developmental/general and technical/specific frameworks are well known and have heuristic value, formal interventions are few and far between,[9,22] although some exist in family medicine.[62]

Institutions known for substantial FD programs use systematic approaches. In addition to the AAMC, POD, and AMEE, these include the University of Toronto Centre for Faculty Development, which uses programs for best education in practice, education scholarship, research in education, and interprofessional education; the Staff Development Centre of Maastricht University; the University of Massachusetts Medical School; and the Harvard Macy Institute. Practices include a multifaceted mentoring program,[63] structured annual faculty reviews,[64] faculty incentives for academic productivity,[65] and efforts to translate promotion criteria.[66] Other fine innovations in medical psychiatric education are teaching academies[67] and intramural grant programs,[68] as well as a centralized unit, office, committee, program, and/or cooperative. More focused efforts have been related to individual consultation, university-wide initiatives (eg, orientation, workshop), intensive seminars, grants/award incentives, and resource guides/publications.[22] Outcomes grounded in values, priorities, and practices are needed to align methods, evaluation, quality improvement, and other processes.[69,70]

AHCs have traditionally emphasized research careers and assessed progress based on funding. Successful research careers depend on many factors, particularly a desire for and commitment to high-quality research, theme-specific publications, progressive grants, research guidance, and willingness to spend the time required coupled with learning from and withstanding failure.[71] A review of 19 articles, with no prospective studies, showed that mentoring and guided and participatory learning were the most successful enabling mechanisms.[72] Other best practices included niche assessment, research literacy, skills/competencies, a collaborative learning/education environment, meaningful incentives, access to/allocation of resources, grant/research partners/teams, internal/external training opportunities, and support from institutional leadership. Common methods include mentoring (both general/developmental and technical/specific), workshops, online resources, in-person short courses, in-depth seminar series, intensive multiday extramural training programs, and grant prereview programs.[73]

Medicine and higher education have been moving from one-on-one to groups and from cross-sectional training to longitudinal models; these feature team-based, project-based, and interprofessional-based initiatives, framed as PD and professional learning communities.[74,75] These frameworks facilitate collegiality, team role/leader development, authentic learning in the workplace, socialization, and attitude/motivation change; flexibility, management of setbacks/delays, and other adjustments are featured. These relationships increase socialization, reduce isolation and promote shared goals; they also change attitudes toward organizations, provide skills and knowledge, and adjust leadership behaviors in faculty.[23] A framework for FD in continuing interprofessional education and collaborative practice is built on best practices, experience in its delivery, and evaluation to promote capacity for dissemination of concepts relating to interprofessional education and interprofessional collaboration in health care environments.[76] These efforts enhance interprofessional collaboration, patient care, and health outcomes via curricula, role modeling, and strategic planning.

Other key areas are leadership, workforce development, and business administration.[60] Based on trends discussed earlier, leaders are needed with skills in facilitating groups, communicating institutional goals, and leveraging resources. For example, research and teaching skill development is an investment has measurable impact on faculty careers.[77] Other leadership programs feature group mentoring, feedback, and integration of early career faculty into the community, and individual skill development, academic planning, and networking.[78] Broadly, though, it is important to build the team right from the start when possible,[79] hire for attitude and train for skill,[80] and to understand life cycle issues of organizational growth and team development.[81] Communication, conflict resolution techniques, a process to build trust, and joint problem solving are suggested.[82] For psychiatrists, it is too tempting to get into the "why" of issues, rather than helping people identify behaviors/actions to change/adapt.[83] The role of conflict identification and management is particularly key in sustaining community collaboration.[84]

Programs by Executive Leadership in Academic Medicine (ELAM) and AAMC and for women's leadership have had some impact and provide a possible prototype for other specific programs.[85] The AAMC survey of a national cohort of 2779 of career development programs (eg, early-career and midcareer women in medicine seminars, ELAM) were asked about 16 skills (ie, newly acquired, improved, or not improved).[86] Four skills predominated across all 3 programs: interpersonal skills, leadership, negotiation, and networking. The skills that attendees endorsed differed by respondents' career stages, more so than by program attended. In the short term, institutions are targeting specific skills (eg, negotiation) to make progress.[87]

Diversity initiatives in PD are moving quickly, at least in terms of guides and resources, but implementation, evaluation, and impact take patience because of the complexity. The AAMC's Diversity Research Forum, 2008, focused on recruitment, retention, and promotion. The AAMC's Striving Toward Excellence Faculty Diversity in Medical Education Report, 2009, has essentials (eg, Diversity and Inclusion Guide; Assessing Culture and Climate) and specifics (eg, Curricular and Institutional Climate Changes to Improve Health Care for Individuals Who Are LGBT, Gender Nonconforming, or Born with DSD [disorder of sex development]).[88,89] There is great effort in aligning the physicians of today with the population of today, such that recruitment and retention of students, residents, and faculty is key.[90] There is a question about how best to tangibly shift committee membership, name heads of searches, and integrate leaders,[91] although recruitment of diverse medical students pushes faculty recruitments.[92] Accordingly, the AAMC is evaluating cultural competence education and training related to diversity efforts.[93]

DISCUSSION

Overall, there are many PD or FD best practices,[8,9,23,24] including mentoring, teaching academies, MD/PhD and early career award programs, and those specialized for groups (eg, women, underrepresented minorities). Institutions have traditionally relied on formal mentoring related to academic productivity in medicine, but even outcomes from highly structured and well-mentored MD/PhD and early career award programs for research fall short of expectations.[29] Psychosocial and/or interpersonal functions, which have been referred to as informal mentoring, have been overlooked[94] but are crucial for faculty satisfaction, self-efficacy, socialization,[38] and retention.[95] A challenge, though, is to approach PD conceptually but personalize the enterprise for individual faculty, groups, departments, and institutions.

The best businesses use customized but systematic approaches to tackle difficult long-term goals like PD, because they want to keep their human capital.[96–98] These efforts take into account industry competition and projections on demographic, sociocultural, political/legal, technology, economic, and global factors and trends (eg, Porter's[99] Five-Forces model).[76] Relationships are critical in sharing and leveraging knowledge and in acquiring resources (known as social capital) through the network of relationships throughout the organization and extending to relationships between the company and its suppliers, customers, and partners. The model includes an environmental analysis by managers to evaluate or reevaluate biases, assumptions, and presuppositions internally, as well as about the industry, making money, the competition, and the customers.[80]

With the workforce changing because of generational differences, it is important to create a stimulating, rewarding environment and shared core mission/values where people want to work. When this theory is applied to academic medicine, perhaps the competition is internal; the clinical, teaching, research, service, administrative, and business missions that compete with PD. In medicine, the capital includes the faculty, trainees, interdisciplinary teams (physician, nurse, staff), patients, researchers/scientists, and knowledge and other expertise that they hold. All groups, including patients, become influencers who do not want to disappoint others or lose the trust of others (ie, family, friend, customer, peer, leader). So, building a strong human-to-human relationship distributes the brand and human capital within and across the company; this is the intellectual capital. If the human capital is not productive and happy, the full potential of the organization is not reached and there are problems (eg, attrition). Strategies to improve quality of life are typically intradiscipline (eg, physicians), interdiscipline health (eg, teams of care), and nonhealth interdiscipline (eg, health, finance, janitor).[80]

Success has been measured by wellness and career progression, with alignment of personal values with the organization's culture of academic vitality.[30] Feeling successful and enjoying the work is central to quality of life and vitality and may help to better prevent burnout, suicide, and substance use.[100] Increasing rates of burnout, stress, and disengagement among faculty, residents, students, and practicing physicians have caused alarm in academic medicine, suggesting that the oft-competing are taking a toll on faculty and institutional vitality.[101] Inquiry and a framework for a greater understanding of faculty well-being are needed to understand how vitality is experienced, defined, and modulated in the context of academic medicine. As Dr Thomas Viggiano said at the Harvard Macy Institute in 2004,[102] "Faculty vitality means the ongoing realization of goals ... This is a career-long journey, not a destination." Promoting scholarship in FD requires relevant research paradigms and methodologies (eg, quantitative and qualitative evaluation).[43]

Psychiatric leaders and faculty may provide perspective on the challenging issues related to PD. The profession emphasizes how important it is to explore beliefs, norms, and values as part of a developmental process of growing and making purposeful change. It also emphasizes management of stress and adapting to adverse situations. On one hand, the profession topographically analyzes the smallest detail, and on the other, it tries to keep it simple and practical. The work of Erikson[37] and

Vaillant[36] provides a structure and process to assessment of needs, planning, and diagnosing problems. Maslow's[103] hierarchy of needs, from human developmental psychology, also describes the stages of growth in humans related to behavioral motivation (ie, physiologic, safety, belonging and love, esteem, and self-actualization).[103] Nonetheless, if clinicians (only) try to think their way through it, rather than live or actualize it, they become prone to the same bad outcomes. Well-being and happiness are generally part of a rewarding career, and physicians work best when they take care of themselves and feel supported.[100]

Diversity initiatives are increasing to remedy several issues and may be an indicator of broader institutional malaise. Surveys of women leaders suggest that there is (1) a wide variation in gender climate; (2) lack of parity in rank and leadership; (3) lack of retention; (4) lack of gender equity in compensation; and (5) a disproportionate burden of family responsibilities and work-life challenges for career progression.[104] Although increases in diverse faculty are being seen, programs do not always effect change.[105] Change in medical education institutions requires significant effort, such that the Royal College of Physicians and Surgeons is introducing the Competence by Design (CBD) FD initiative, which emphasizes that faculty first have to understand, design, and engage in the change in order to later model and teach it.[106]

Activities that bring people together to explore values, engage others to feel included, and empower faculty with leadership at every level help both faculty and the organization to shift workplace culture. O'Sullivan and Irby[107] have proposed that FD is most successful when there is an emphasis on the power of communities of teaching practice and networks of relationships for supporting and strengthening instruction in the workplace. Diversity of knowledge and skills contributes to a creative team process, and innovation emanates from a group process that is open, encourages new ideas, and promotes reflection. A PD culture as part of the educational mission contributes to the institution's task-related skills, information, perspectives, and ultimately creativity.[108]

SUMMARY

PD refers to training, formal education, and/or advanced professional learning intended to help clinicians, teachers, researchers, and administrators improve their professional knowledge, competence, skill, and effectiveness. Like other parts of medicine, progress may be accomplished by a systematic needs assessment of key partners (ie, faculty, departments, institutions, national organizations), intervention, monitoring, and evaluation/quality improvement. Institutions, despite many priorities, constraints, and other challenges, must focus on the wellness, vitality, and initiative of faculty and other leaders in both psychiatry and medicine. Inquiry, engagement, and inclusion in the process and meeting concrete FD needs are suggested. Multidimensional approaches, including mentoring and socialization, are suggested. Interprofessional, team-based, and project-based longitudinal initiatives provide support, learning opportunities, promote socialization, build a positive workplace culture, and provide a venue for educational innovation. More research is needed on design, implementation, and outcomes for PD.

ACKNOWLEDGMENTS

The authors would like to acknowledge the American Association of Directors of Psychiatry Residency Training, the American Directors of Medical Student Education in Psychiatry, and the Association For Academic Psychiatry.

REFERENCES

1. Armstrong EG, Mackey M, Spear SJ. Medical education as a process management problem. Acad Med 2004;79(8):721–8.

2. Institute of Medicine. Crossing the quality chasm: a new health system for the 21st century. Washington, DC: National Academic Press; 2001. Available at: https://doi.org/10.17226/10027. Accessed December 27, 2018.

3. Institute of Medicine. The core competencies needed for healthcare professionals. Health professions education: a bridge to quality. Washington, DC: The National Academies Press; 2003. https://doi.org/10.17226/10681. Available at: http://www.nationalacademies.org/hmd/Reports/2003/Health-Professions-Education-A-Bridge-to-Quality.aspx. Accessed December 27, 2018.

4. Wallace S, May SA. Assessing and enhancing quality through outcomes-based continuing professional development (CPD): a review of current practice. Vet Rec 2016;179(20):515–20.

5. Opperman C, Liebig D, Bowling J, et al. Measuring return on investment for professional development activities: 2018 Updates. J Nurses Prof Dev 2018;34(6): 303–12.

6. Cervero RM, Gaines JK. Accreditation Council for continuing medical education effectiveness of continuing medical education. 2018. Updated Synthesis of Systematic Reviews. Available at: http://www.accme.org/sites/default/files/652_20141104_Effectiveness_of_Continuing_Medical_Education_Cervero_and_Gaines.pdf. Accessed December 27, 2018.

7. Centra JA. Types of faculty development programs. J High Educ 1978;49(2): 151–62.

8. Bland CJ, Schmitz CC, Stritter FT, et al. Successful faculty in academic medicine: essential skills and how to acquire them. New York: Springer; 1990.

9. Steinert YG. Faculty development in the health professions. New York: Springer; 2014. p. 3–25.

10. Swanwick T, McKimm J. Faculty development for leadership and management. In: Steinert YG, editor. Faculty development in the health professions. New York: Springer; 2014. p. 53–78.

11. Thomas A, Steinert Y. Knowledge translation and faculty development: from theory to practice. In: Steinert YG, editor. Faculty development in the health professions. New York: Springer; 2014. p. 399–418.

12. Association of American Medical Colleges. Retention of full-time clinical MD Faculty at US Medical Schools, February 2011, AAMC Analysis in Brief. Available at: https://www.aamc.org/download/175974/data/aibvol11_no2.pdf. Accessed December 27, 2018.

13. Steinert Y, Mann K, Anderson B, et al. A systematic review of faculty development initiatives designed to enhance teaching effectiveness: a 10-year update: BEME Guide No. 40. Med Teach 2016;38(8):769–86.

14. American Association of Medical Colleges. The strategic imperative: leading change to improve health. 2018. Available at: https://www.aamc.org/about/strategicpriorities/. Accessed December 27, 2018.

15. Gillespie KJ, Robertson DL. Professional and organizational development higher education network. San Francisco (CA): Jossey-Bass; 2010.

16. Association for Medical Education in Europe (AMEE). Available at: https://amee.org/amee-committees/faculty-development. Accessed December 27, 2018.

17. Hilty DM, Srinivasan M, Xiong G, et al. Lessons from psychiatry and psychiatric education for medical learners and teachers. Int Rev Psychiatry 2013;25: 329–37.

18. Engle GL. The clinical application of the biopsychosocial model. Am J Psychiatry 1980;137(5):535–44.

19. Baker VL. Success after tenure: supporting mid-career faculty. Sterling (VA): Stylus Publishing; 2019.

20. Westberg J, Jason H. The enhancement of teaching skills in US medical schools: an overview and some recommendations. Med Teach 1981;3(3):100–4.

21. Tiberius RG. A brief history of educational development: implications for teachers and developers. In: Lieberman D, Wehlberg C, editors. To improve the academy, vol. 20. Bolton (MA): Resources for faculty, instructional, and organizational development; 2002. p. 20–37. Anker.

22. Sorcinelli MD, Austin AE, Eddy PL, et al. Creating the future of faculty development. San Francisco (CA): Jossey-Bass; 2006. p. 1–28.

23. Steinert Y, Naismith L, Mann K. Faculty development initiatives designed to promote leadership in medical education. A BEME systematic review: BEME Guide No. 19. Med Teach 2012;34(6):483–503.

24. Leslie K, Baker L, Egan-Lee E, et al. Advancing faculty development in medical education: a systematic review. Acad Med 2013;88(7):1038–45.

25. Roberts LW, Hilty DM. Handbook of career development in academic psychiatry and behavioral sciences, second edition. Washington, DC: American Psychiatric Publishing Incorporated; 2017.

26. Hilty DM, Yager J, Seritan A, et al. A historical review of key events and components of faculty/professional development in psychiatry. Psych Clin N Amer, in press.

27. Sheets KJ, Schwenk TL. Faculty development for family medicine educators: an agenda for future activities. Teach Learn Med 1990;2(3):141–8.

28. Schofield SJ, Bradley S, Macrae C, et al. How we encourage faculty development. Med Teach 2010;32(11):883–6.

29. Marsh JD, Todd RF 3rd. Training and sustaining physician scientists: what is success? Am J Med 2015;128(4):431–6.

30. Leslie K. Faculty development for academic and career development. In: Steinert YG, editor. Faculty development in the health professions. New York: Springer; 2014. p. 97–118.

31. Royal College of Physicians and Surgeons of Canada. A continuing commitment to lifelong learning: a concise guide to maintenance of certification. 2011. Available at: http://www.royalcollege.ca/portal/page/portal/rc/common/documents/moc_program/moc_short_guide_e.pdf. Accessed December 27, 2018.

32. Pratt DD. Five perspectives on teaching in adult and higher education. Malabar (FL): Krieger Publishing; 1998.

33. Kolb D. Experiential learning: experience as the source of learning and development. Englewood Cliffs (NJ): Prentice-Hall; 1984.

34. Bruffee K. Collaborative learning: higher education, interdependence, and the authority of knowledge. Baltimore (MD): Johns Hopkins University Press; 1999.

35. Clarke D, Hollingsworth H. Elaborating a model of teacher professional growth. Teach Educ 2002;18(8):947–67.

36. Vaillant G. Aging well. Boston: Little, Brown and Co; 2002.

37. Erikson EH. Childhood and society. 2nd edition. New York: Norton; 1963.

38. American Psychiatric Association. Diagnostic and statistical manual of mental disorders. 5th edition. Washington, DC: American Psychiatric Press, Incorporated; 2013.

39. Shollen SL, Bland CJ, Center BA, et al. Relating mentor type and mentoring behaviors to academic medicine faculty satisfaction and productivity at one medical school. Acad Med 2014;89(9):1267–75.

40. Canadian Institutes of Health Research. More about knowledge translation at CIHR: knowledge translation – definition. 2012. Available at: http://www.cihr-irsc.gc.ca/e/39033.html. Accessed December 27, 2018.

41. Davis D, Evans M, Jadad A, et al. The case for knowledge translation: Shortening the journey from evidence to effect. BMJ 2003;327(7405):33–5.

42. Glasgow RE, Lichtenstein E, Marcus AC. Why don't we see more translation of health promotion research to practice? Rethinking the efficacy-to-effectiveness transition. Am J Public Health 2003;93(8):1261–7.

43. O'Sullivan P, Irby DM. Promoting scholarship in faculty development: relevant research paradigms and methodologies. In: Steinert YG, editor. Faculty development in the health professions. New York: Springer; 2014. p. 375–98.

44. Hilty DM, Uno J, Torous J, et al. Role of technology in faculty development in psychiatry. Psych Clin N Amer, in press.

45. Office of Educational Technology. Reimagining the role of technology in education: 2017 National Education Technology Plan Update, Higher Education Supplement. 2017. Available at: https://tech.ed.gov/files/2017/01/NETP17.pdf. Accessed December 27, 2018.

46. Levy F, Murnane RJ. A role for technology in professional development? Lessons from IBM. Phi Delta Kappan 2004;85(10):728–34.

47. Matzen NJ, Edmunds JA. Technology as a catalyst for change. J Res Tech Educ 2007;39(4):417–30.

48. Hilty DM, Crawford A, Teshima J, et al. A framework for telepsychiatric training and e-health: competency-based education, evaluation and implications. Int Rev Psychiatry 2015;27(6):569–92.

49. Maheu MM, Drude KP, Hertlein KM, et al. An interprofessional framework for telebehavioral health competencies. J Tech Behav Sci 2018;3(2):108–40.

50. Hilty DM, Zalpuri I, Stubbe D, et al. Social media/networking and psychiatric education: competencies, teaching methods, and implications. J Tech Behav Sci 2018;19:722.

51. Zalpuri I, Liu HY, Stubbe D, et al. Social media and networking competencies for psychiatric education: skills, teaching methods, and implications. Acad Psychiatry 2018;42(6):808–17.

52. Hilty DM, Chan S, Torous, J, et al. A competency-based framework for psych/behavioral health apps for trainees, faculty, programs and health systems. Psych Clin N Amer, in press.

53. Lieff SJ. Faculty development: yesterday, today and tomorrow: guide supplement 33.2 – Viewpoint. Med Teach 2010;32(5):429–31.

54. Srinivasan M, Li ST, Meyers FJ, et al. Teaching as a competency for medical educators: competencies for medical educators. Acad Med 2011;86(10):1211–20.

55. Kirch DG. The role of academic psychiatry in the transformation of health care. Acad Psychiatry 2011;35(2):73–5.

56. Blitzstein S, Seritan A, Sockalingham S, et al. From industry to generativity: the first twelve years of the Association for Academic Psychiatry Master Educator Program. Acad Psychiatry 2016;40(4):576–83.

57. De Golia SG, Cagande CC, Ahn MS, et al. Faculty development for teaching faculty in psychiatry: where we are and what we need. Acad Psychiatry 2018. https://doi.org/10.1007/s40596-018-0916-4.

58. Mellman LA. Cultivating careers in the American Association of Directors of Psychiatric Residency Training. Acad Psychiatry 2007;31(2):101–2.

59. Sierles FS. The association of directors of medical student education in psychiatry. Acad Psychiatry 2007;31(2):107–9.

60. Lieff S, Banack JG, Baker L, et al. Understanding the needs of department chairs in academic medicine. Acad Med 2013;88(7):960–6.

61. Pololi LH, Dennis K, Winn GM, et al. A needs assessment of medical school faculty: caring for the caretakers. J Contin Educ Health Prof 2003;23:21–9.

62. Simpson D, Marcdante K, Morzinski J, et al. Fifteen years of aligning faculty development with primary care clinician–educator roles and academic advancement at the Medical College of Wisconsin. Acad Med 2006;81: 945–53. Available at: http://journals.lww.com/ academicmedicine/Fulltext/ 2006/11000/ Fifteen_Years_of_Aligning_Faculty_ Development_With.4.aspx. Accessed December 27, 2018.

63. Chen MM, Sandborg CI, Hudgins L, et al. a multifaceted mentoring program for junior faculty in academic pediatrics. Teach Learn Med 2016;28(3):320–8.

64. Robboy SJ, McLendon R. Structured annual faculty review program accelerates professional development and promotion: long-term experience of the Duke University Medical Center's pathology department. Acad Pathol 2017;4. 2374289516689471.

65. Hales RE, Shahrokh NC, Servis M. A progress report on a department of psychiatry faculty practice plan designed to reward educational and research productivity. Acad Psychiatry 2009;33(3):248–51.

66. Hilty DM, Callahan EJ. Understanding and preparing for the process of academic promotion. In: Roberts LW, Hilty DM, editors. Handbook of career development in academic psychiatry and behavioral sciences. 2nd edition. Washington, DC: American Psychiatric Publishing Incorporated; 2017. p. 141–60.

67. Muller JH, Irby DM. Developing educational leaders: the teaching scholars program at the University of California, San Francisco, School of Medicine. Acad Med 2006;81:959–64. Available at: http://journals.lww.com/ academicmedicine/ Fulltext/2006/11000/ Developing_Educational_Leaders The_ Teaching.6.aspx. Accessed December 27, 2018.

68. Adler SR, Chang A, Loeser H, et al. The impact of intramural grants on educators' careers and on medical education innovation. Acad Med 2015;90(6): 827–31.

69. Harden RM, Crosby JR, Davis MH. AMEE guide no. 14: outcome-based education: part 1-An introduction to outcome-based education. Med Teach 1999; 21:7–14.

70. Miller G. The assessment of clinical skills/competence/performance. Acad Med 1990;65(Suppl):S63–7.

71. Gail Neely J, Smith RJ, Graboyes EM, et al. Guide to academic research career development. Laryngoscope Investig Otolaryngol 2016;1(1):19–24.

72. Teruya SA, Bazargan-Hejazi S, Mojtahedzadeh M, et al. A review of programs, components and outcomes in biomedical research faculty development. Int J Univ Teach Fac Dev 2013;4(4):223–36.

73. Baldwin CD, Goldblum RM, Rassin DK, et al. Facilitating faculty development and research through critical review of grant proposals and articles. Acad Med 1994;69(1):62–4.
74. Mennin S, Kalishman S, Eklund M, et al. Project-based faculty development by international health professions educators: practical strategies. Med Teach 2013;35:e971–7.
75. Gast I, Schildkamp K, van der Veen JT. Team-based professional development interventions in higher education: a systematic review. Rev Educ Res 2017; 87(4):736–67.
76. Silver IL, Leslie K. Faculty development for continuing interprofessional education and collaborative practice. J Contin Educ Health Prof 2017;37(4):262–7.
77. Gruppen LD, Frohna AZ, Anderson RM, et al. Faculty development for educational leadership and scholarship. Acad Med 2003;78(2):137–41.
78. Wingard DL, Garman KA, Reznik V. Facilitating faculty success: outcomes and cost benefit of the UCSD National Center of Leadership in Academic Medicine. Acad Med 2004;79(10Suppl):S9–11.
79. Dye CF. Leadership in healthcare: essential values and skills. 2nd edition. Chicago: Health Administration Press; 2010.
80. Kamath R. Strategic management. New York: McGraw-Hill; 2014.
81. Coppola MN. Leveraging team building strategies. Making strategies work to an organization's advantage. Healthc Exec 2008;23(3):70, 72-73.
82. Mohr J, Spekman R. Characteristics of partnership success: Partnership attributes, communication behavior, and conflict resolution techniques. Strat Manag J 1994;15(2):135–52.
83. Talbott JA, Hales RE. Textbook of administrative psychiatry: new concepts for changing a behavioral health system. 2nd edition. Washington, DC: American Psychiatric Press, Incorporated; 2001.
84. Blanch AK, Boustead R, Boothroyd RA, et al. The role of conflict identification and management in sustaining community collaboration: Report on a four-year exploratory study. J Behav Health Serv Res 2015;42(3):324–33.
85. Bickel J, Wara D, Atkinson BF, et al, Association of American Medical Colleges Project Implementation Committee. Increasing women's leadership in academic medicine: report of the AAMC Project Implementation Committee. Acad Med 2002;77(10):1043–61.
86. Helitzer DL, Newbill SL, Morahan PS, et al. Perceptions of skill development of participants in three national career development programs for women faculty in academic medicine. J Womens Health (Larchmt) 2016;25(4):360–70.
87. Levine RB, González-Fernández M, Bodurtha J, et al. Implementation and evaluation of the Johns Hopkins University School of Medicine leadership program for women faculty. J Womens Health (Larchmt) 2015;24(5):360–6.
88. Association of American Medical Colleges. Diversity research forum. 2008. Available at: https://members.aamc.org/eweb/upload/The%20Diversity%20 Research%20Forum%20The%20Importance%20and%20Benefits%20of%20 Diverse%20Fac%20in%20Acad%20Med.pdf.
89. Association of American Medical Colleges. Striving toward excellence faculty diversity in medical education report. 2009. Available at: https://members.aamc. org/eweb/upload/Striving%20Towards%20Excellect%20Faculty%20Diversity%20 in%20Med%20Ed.pdf.
90. Rodriguez JE, Campbell KM, Fogarty JP, et al. Underrepresented minority faculty in academic medicine: a systematic review of URM faculty development. Fam Med 2014;46(2):100–4.

91. Nivet MA. A diversity 3.0 update: are we moving the needle enough? Acad Med 2015;90(12):1591–3.
92. Page KR, Castillo-Page L, Wright SM. Faculty diversity programs in U.S. medical schools and characteristics associated with higher faculty diversity. Acad Med 2011;86(10):1221–8.
93. Association of American Medical Colleges. Evaluating cultural competence education and training. 2015. Available at: https://www.aamc.org/download/427350/data/.
94. Kram KE. Mentoring at work: developmental relationships in organizational life. Glenview (IL): Scott Foresman; 1985.
95. Allen TD, Eby LT. Factors related to mentor reports of mentoring functions provided: gender and relational characteristics. Sex Roles 2004;50:129–39.
96. Cleveland Clinic. Video on empathy. 2018. Available at: http://www.youtube.com/watch?v=cDDWvj_q-o8&feature=youtu.be. Accessed December 27, 2018.
97. Cosgrove T. The concepts behind Cleveland Clinic's success. Becker Hospital Review. 2014. Available at: https://www.beckershospitalreview.com/hospital-management-administration/dr-toby-cosgrove-the-concepts-behind-cleveland-clinic-s-success.html. Accessed December 27, 2018.
98. Tobak S. 10 Secrets to Trader Joe's Success. 2010. Available at: https://www.cbsnews.com/news/10-secrets-to-trader-joes-success/. Accessed December 27, 2018.
99. Porter ME. How competitive forces shape strategy. Harv Bus Rev 1979;59(2):137–45.
100. Corbett BA, Marla V, Nanda N, et al. Taking care of yourself. In: Roberts LW, Hilty DM, editors. Handbook of career development in academic psychiatry and behavioral sciences. 2nd edition. Washington, DC: American Psychiatric Publishing Incorporated; 2017. p. 373–84.
101. Shah DT, Williams VN, Thorndyke LE, et al. Restoring faculty vitality in academic medicine when burnout threatens. Acad Med 2018;93(7):979–84.
102. Viggiano TR, Strobel HW. The Career Management Life Cycle: A Model for Supporting and Sustaining Faculty Vitality and Wellness. In: Cole TH, Goodrich TJ, Gritz ER, editors. Faulty health in Academic Medicine Physicians, Scientists, and the Pressures of Success. New York: Springer; 2009. p. 73–81.
103. Maslow AH. A theory of human motivation. Psychol Rev 1943;50(4):370–96.
104. Carr PL, Gunn CM, Kaplan SA, et al. Inadequate progress for women in academic medicine: findings from the National Faculty Study. J Womens Health (Larchmt) 2015;24(3):190–9.
105. Guevara JP, Adanga E, Avakame E, et al. Minority faculty development programs and underrepresented minority faculty representation at US Medical Schools. JAMA 2013;310(21):2297–304.
106. Royal College of Physicians and Surgeons of Canada. Competence by Design (CBD). Available at: http://www.royalcollege.ca/rcsite/cbd/cbd-faculty-development-e. Accessed December 27, 2018.
107. O'Sullivan PS, Irby DM. Reframing research on faculty development. Acad Med 2011;86(4):421–8.
108. West MA. Sparkling fountains or stagnant ponds: an integrated model of creativity and innovation implementation in work groups. Appl Psychol: An Int Rev 2002;51(3). Available at: https://doi.org/10.1111/1464-0597.00951. Accessed May 1, 2019.

A Historical Review of Key Events and Components of Faculty and Professional Development in Psychiatry

Donald M. Hilty, MD, MBA[a],*, Joel Yager, MD[b],
Andreea L. Seritan, MD[c], Ruth Levine, MD[d],
Sandra M. DeJong, MD, MSc[e], Jonathan Borus, MD[f,1]

KEYWORDS

- Faculty • Development • Psychiatry • Apprentice • Organization • Profession
- Career • History

KEY POINTS

- Faculty development is instrumental for enhancing the vitality of individual careers and the advancement of the profession as a whole.
- Faculty development occurs in several ways, beginning with 1:1 apprenticeships and mentorships, peer networking, and via formal organizational programs.
- National organizations have provided structures for increasing faculty development efforts nationally and internationally.

INTRODUCTION

The evolution of psychiatry coupled with parallel evolutions in biology, psychology, social sciences, business, education and health care systems, provides the shifting contexts in which faculty development (FD) in psychiatry continues to occur. A

Disclosure Statement: The authors have nothing to disclose.
[a] Mental Health, Northern California Veterans Administration Health Care System, Department of Psychiatry and Behavioral Sciences, University of California Davis, 10535 Hospital Way, Mather, CA 95655, USA; [b] Department of Psychiatry, University of Colorado School of Medicine, MC A011-04, 13001 East 17th Place, Aurora, CO 80045, USA; [c] Department of Psychiatry, University of California, San Francisco, UCSF Weill Institute for Neurosciences, 401 Parnassus Avenue, Box 0984-APC, San Francisco, CA 94143, USA; [d] Department of Psychiatry and Behavioral Sciences, Student Affairs and Admissions, School of Medicine, University of Texas Medical Branch, Ashbel Smith Building, Suite 1.210. 301 University Boulevard, Galveston, TX 77555-1307, USA; [e] Department of Psychiatry, Cambridge Health Alliance, Harvard University School of Medicine, Cambridge Hospital, 1493 Cambridge Street, Cambridge, MA 02139, USA; [f] Brigham and Women's Hospital, Harvard Medical School
[1] Present address: 48 Avondale Road, Newton, MA 02459.
* Corresponding author.
E-mail addresses: donh032612@gmail.com; Donald.Hilty@va.gov

Psychiatr Clin N Am 42 (2019) 357–373
https://doi.org/10.1016/j.psc.2019.05.001
0193-953X/19/© 2019 Elsevier Inc. All rights reserved.

pivotal issue is how we pass on psychiatry's current identity, values, attitudes, and skills to current and future generations—and continue to reflect on and create our evolving values.[1,2] Up to the mid 20th century, early career faculty learned what they needed to do largely by muddling through (still a favorite coping mechanism),[3] based on apprenticeship and developmental perspectives.[4] Those fortunate enough to be able to access generous local mentors in their home institutions learned what these mentors had to teach. Often, these lessons were limited to what each relatively small group of mentors knew, so that the perspectives, attitudes, and skills transmitted in this fashion were somewhat restricted. However, faculty attrition caused significant discontinuities and replacement costs have been significant.[5]

In the 1960s, the emergence of several larger professional communities spurred new possibilities affecting psychiatric FD, impacting clinician-educators and researchers (**Table 1**). These emerging structures stemmed from both top-down (eg, National Institute of Mental Health [NIMH] Career Teachers) and bottom-up events (eg, movements toward pedagogy by the Association for Academic Psychiatry [AAP]). In the 1970sand 1980s, FD resources for clinician educators were further enhanced as the American Psychiatric Association (APA) Office of Education brought academic organizations together. These efforts provided important assets to early career faculty: increased access to mentors and peers across the country; rapid access to information about new and emerging trends, regulations, and opportunities; and advanced training opportunities through seminars, workshops, courses, lectures, and even formalized certificate programs.[6]

Still, there are few generally accepted best practices or well-studied, longitudinal approaches to FD, and there has been little evaluation/research of FD initiatives in medicine globally, and even less so in psychiatry.[7–10] Although the importance for FD is often acknowledged, time and financial resources allocated to FD is usually quite limited in most departments and institutions, which are largely focused on other priorities (**Fig. 1**).[11] Fortunately, several organizations play pivotal roles by promoting FD directly (eg, AAP) and/or via training missions (eg, American Association of Directors of Psychiatric Residency Training [AADPRT], Association of Directors of Medical Student Education in Psychiatry [ADMSEP]).[12–14] The need for advanced FD (eg, for leadership skill development for positions aspiring chairs and deans) has been increasingly recognized as well.

Too important to be left to chance, FD should be approached systematically.[15] Accordingly, this article offers historical perspectives and outlines fundamental structures and processes that inform FD related to clinical care, research, and training. It also highlights key FD contributions from academic organizations in psychiatry, focusing on faculty and career development in psychiatry. Other important aspects of professional development, academic affairs/personnel and accreditation (eg, Accreditation Council of Graduate Medical Education [ACGME], Liaison Committee on Medical Education) are discussed in companion article in this edition.

FACULTY DEVELOPMENT: HOW CLINICIANS, PROGRAMS, AND OTHER INITIATIVES CARRY THE FIELD OF PSYCHIATRY FORWARD

Our values, attitudes, and best practices continue to evolve both from the top down, through our national leadership organizations, and from the bottom up, through the efforts of psychiatrists, interprofessional colleagues, patients, and communities. As new science expands our view, we are continuously challenged clinically, ethically, and in

Table 1
Key historical developments in psychiatry and medicine

Time Period	Event
1600s–1800s	
1656	Pitié-Salpêtrière Hospital in Paris opens
1783	Bicêtre Hospital, Paris, for the "mentally defective," Chains removed from patients
1808	German physician Johann Christian Reil used the term "psychiatry"
1812	Benjamin Rush advocates for humane treatment for the mentally ill in *Medical Inquiries and Observations Upon Diseases of the Mind*, the first American textbook on psychiatry
1844	American Psychiatric Association founded
1847	American Medical Association founded
1887	National Institutes of Health founded
1893	German psychiatrist Emil Kraepelin clinically defined dementia praecox, later reformulated as schizophrenia
1895	Sigmund Freud and Josef Breuer, Austria, *Studies on Hysteria*
1895	"How soon can a child go mad?" by Harold Maudsley, *Pathology of the Mind*
1900s	
1900–1930s	Classical conditioning (Pavlov), operant conditioning (Skinner)
1902	Adolf Meyer became director of the New York State Psychiatric Institute: medical model, records and "common sense"
1905	Binet-Simon test, the first intelligence test
1908	Paul Eugene Bleuler, Switzerland, uses the term "schizophrenia"
1911	American Psychoanalytic Association founded
1913	Carl Jung, analytical psychology
1917	Object relations theory, with Ferenczi and later British psychologists Melanie Klein, Donald Winnicott, 1940s and 1950s
1920	Hermann Rorschach developed the Rorschach Inkblot Test
1927	Julius Wagner-Jauregg, Austrian psychiatrist, Nobel Prize in Physiology or Medicine, 1927, therapeutic value of malaria inoculation in the treatment of dementia paralytica
1927	Manfred Sakel, Austrian psychiatrist, insulin shock therapy as a treatment for psychosis; discontinued in 1970s
1932	Jean Piaget, cognitive theory, publication of his work *The Moral Judgment of Children*
1934	The American Board of Psychiatry and Neurology, Inc., founded
1938	Italian neurologist Ugo Cerletti and Italian psychiatrist Dr Lucio Bini discovered electroconvulsive therapy
1942	American Psychosomatic Society founded Carl Rogers, client-centered therapy
1946	National Mental Health Act, funding for National Institute of Mental Health, out of concern for public and Veterans
1947	António Egas Moniz, Nobel Prize, 1949 for his discovery of the therapeutic value of leucotomy in certain psychoses
1948	Lithium carbonate's ability to stabilize mood demonstrated by Australian psychiatrist John Cade, first effective medicine for the treatment of mental illness

(continued on next page)

Table 1 (continued)	
Time Period	**Event**
1949	National Institute of Mental Health established and funding for children in 1970s
1950	The World Psychiatric Association was founded
1952	The American Psychiatric Association published the first *Diagnostic and Statistical Manual of Mental Disorders*; revised in 1968, 1980/7, 1994, 2000, and 2013
1953	American Academy of Child & Adolescent Psychiatry founded Academy for Consultation-Liaison Psychiatry (formerly Academy of Psychosomatic Medicine) founded
1954	Abraham Maslow, "Motivation and Personality" and hierarchy of needs
1950s–1970s	First monoamine oxidase inhibitor, antipsychotic and benzodiazepine developed Developmental psychology flourished after World War I with Jean Piaget (Switzerland), Lev Vygotsky (Russia), and John Bowlby (UK) Telepsychiatry (video) launches
1960s	Aaron T. Beck developed cognitive therapy
1963	Community Mental Health Centers Act
1956	National Institute of Mental Health founded the Career Teachers Program
1963	American College of Psychiatrists founded
1967	National Institute of Mental Health began independent of the National Institute of Health
1970	American Association of Directors of Psychiatric Residency Training founded
1970	Society for Academic Psychiatry founded; became the Association for Academic Psychiatry in 1971
1974	Association of Directors of Medical Student Education in Psychiatry founded
1977	Biopsychosocial model was proposed by George L. Engel
1977	President Jimmy Carter's Presidential Commission on Mental Health
1977	The *International Classification of Diseases-9* was published by the World Health Organization
1980s	Handheld phone hits market
1981	National Alliance for Research on Schizophrenia and Depression
1990	Mental Health America advocates for Americans with Disabilities Act
1990s	Modern telepsychiatry launches
1994	The Mental Health Parity Act by President Clinton American Psychiatric Association *Outline for Cultural Formulation in Diagnostic and Statistical Manual*
1996	The *International Classification of Diseases-10* was published by the World Health Organization
2000s	
2000	Eric R. Kandel, Nobel Prize in Physiology or Medicine, for their discoveries concerning signal transduction in the nervous system
2000	Genetic researchers map human genes with the aim of isolating the individual chromosome responsible for mental dysfunction
2003	President's (Clinton) New Freedom Commission on Mental Health, Achieving the Promise: Transforming Mental Health Care in America
2008	Mental Health Parity Act

(continued on next page)

Table 1 (*continued*)	
Time Period	**Event**
2010	The Patient Protection and Affordable Care Act (P.L. 111–148; health care reform law signed by President Obama)
2012	Brian K. Kobilka, Stanford University, Nobel Prize in Chemistry, 2012, the communication system between G-protein coupled receptors and body
2013	*Diagnostic and Statistical Manual of Mental Disorders*-5 published
2014	John O'Keefe, May-Britt Moser, and Edvard Moser, Nobel Prize, cells that constitute a positioning system in the brain key to memory

other ways. Creative aspects of our profession are reflected by the many available career options, perspectives about life experiences, and theoretic approaches to treatments. Our varied perspectives on who we are and what we do, contribute to the creative processes forming the face of psychiatry. While advocating for many, we have reduced stigmatization, increased access to care, and helped others in medicine, despite poor remuneration for clinical care (eg, reimbursement via relative value units) and education (ie, most productivity measures do not typically recognize educational contributions).

FD in psychiatry spans clinical, educational, research, and administrative activities[16,17]; several authorities have also included leadership and management.[9] Certain institutions are known for substantial FD programs, usually signified by substantial academic productivity,[18] high rates of medical student recruitment into psychiatry, and/or inter(national) organization leadership. However, limited resources, inadequate

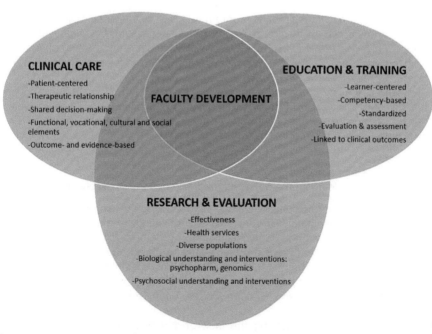

Fig. 1. FD: an intersection of clinical care, education/training, and research/scholarship.

championing, and a lack of systematic approaches in departments and institutions have left many without sufficient support for FD. Another challenge is that faculty interests, roles, and responsibilities change over time, particularly across career stages, suggesting the need for life-long FD.[19] Some institutional competences regarding FD have been suggested, for example, for teaching[20] and for developing telepsychiatric enterprises.[21]

Faculty learn from departmental, institutional, and (inter)national organization experiences in complimentary ways (**Table 2**). Academic organizations such as the AAP, AADPRT, ADMSEP, Association of American Medical Colleges (AAMC), and others have played an increasing role in using new approaches to FD. For example, complex longitudinal FD training models (eg, project-based) require leaders with skills in facilitating groups, communicating institutional goals, and leveraging resources.[22] Distance relationships via technology are also increasing, usually for specific/technical mentoring.

Sophisticated and effective FD sets the stage surpasses simply passing on knowledge, skills, and attitudes—and invites creativity and innovation, inspiring the next generation of psychiatrists and advancing the field through more effective, novel methods of teaching. Psychiatrists must also fully use scientific findings and evidence-based research for care (ie, knowledge translation)[23] and anticipate emerging scientific breakthroughs that will further challenge our ethical principles and impact the skills required to deliver optimal patient care. Ideal FD engages faculty in deep reflection of our core values, and inquiry into what new and effective pedagogical skills will be required to best learn and teach.[24]

KEY DEVELOPMENTS IN PSYCHIATRY: THE NATIONAL INSTITUTE OF MENTAL HEALTH, AMERICAN PSYCHIATRIC ASSOCIATION, AND NATIONAL ACADEMIC ORGANIZATIONS

The NIMH began a career teacher program in 1956, because scholarship, clinical acumen, and research ability did not by themselves necessarily correlate with teaching skill.[25] From the 1960s to the 1980s, nearly all psychiatric department chairs were psychoanalysts, and the NIMH was just starting to conduct and fund biological research. At that time the NIMH also offered a series of training grants for medical schools and residency programs. The program for physician educators was housed within the NIMH's Division of Education, Continuing Education Branch (the equivalent of the nation's center for psychiatric FD of that era) led by Dr Tom Webster. Three funded paths were available:

1. Psychiatry,
2. Residency education, and
3. Family medicine learning mental health and/or retraining in psychiatry.

The NIMH Psychiatric Educator Career Teacher program was led by Dr James Eaton of George Washington University School of Medicine and Health Sciences, who was also tasked with developing education programs for consultation-liaison psychiatrists. These 2-year grant programs were modeled after the NIMH's Career Investigator (research) program. Many notable individuals instrumental in psychiatry's evolution in those decades participated, including Drs Layton McCurdy, Don Lipsitt, Pat McKegney, Carol Nadelson, Braxton McKee, Peter Gruenberg, Lenore Terr, and Ira Glick.

Roughly about 1966, lamenting the lack of a national meeting where career teachers could gather together, Dr McCurdy obtained NIMH funding for several

Table 2
Career development needs: systems and methods responsible for helping faculty meet them

Area of Need	Department	Institution/Health System	(Inter)national Professional Organizations
Career stage			
Early			
Developing professional identity	Peer, team and mentor	Colleagues in medicine	Peer, role model, advisor and/or mentor
Clinical expertise	Service team and/or chief, site/medical director and/or mentor	Workflow, documentation (eg, electronic health record) and other	APA and subspecialty, if applicable
Scholarly expertise	Peer, team with or without group (eg, health services) and mentor; core teaching skills	Adjunct teaching skills, mission (eg, admissions) and interprofessional themes	Continuing medical education, mentor, collaborative groups; journal peer reviewer
Career development	Formal and/or informal via mentor, division leader with or without chair	Seminar, workshop, scholars program (eg, teaching) with or without mentor program; usually cross-sectional	Seminar, workshop with or without mentor program, cross-sectional and/or longitudinal
Wellness	Trainees, peers, services, sites and others	Initiatives to assess, offer resources and intervene, if necessary	Perspective to balance department/institution environment
Mid			
Consolidate professional identity	Supervisor, mentor, educator	Cross-departmental collaboration, interprofessional/interdisciplinary education/mentorship	Long-distance mentor, advisor, sponsor
Clinical expertise	Division chief, vice chair, chair, and/or mentor	Health system administrative leader role	Clinical guidelines/best practices development group member

(continued on next page)

Table 2
(continued)

Area of Need	Department	Institution/Health System	(Inter)national Professional Organizations
Scholarly expertise	Coprincipal/principal investigator on extramural funding, grant proposal reviewer; journal reviewer, editorial board member	Intramural clinical/scholarly/quality improvement proposal reviewer; institution-wide event organizer, chair	Program committee member, chair
Leadership and administrative roles	Mentor, educational/faculty affairs/FD committee member, chair	Core committee chair, associate dean, dean	Mentor, committee chair, professional organization officer, chair
Wellness	Develop service, division, department wellness programs	Disseminate wellness initiatives at local, regional, and national levels	Participate in organizational initiatives to educate/disseminate best practices
Advanced			
Redefine identity	Explore new areas or pursue additional degree, related/unrelated to medicine (MBA, MPH, MS, PhD)	Develop new clinical or educational program/track	Join new organizations, aligned with newly developed interests
Transition to/from leadership positions	Transfer previous knowledge and skills to new process/institution	May change institutions; step down from leadership roles; take on new roles in different areas	Professional organization chair; sponsor and support next generation for leadership roles
Clinical and scholarly expertise	Ongoing FD; educator, mentor, principal investigator - extramural funding	Mentor and sponsor next generation for leadership roles	Clinical guidelines/best practices development group member, chair
Preparing for partial/full retirement	Document programs/guidelines developed, so they can be replicated; succession planning	Succession planning	Succession planning
Wellness	Develop/lead service, division, department wellness programs	Disseminate wellness initiatives at local, regional, and national levels	Lead organizational initiatives to educate/disseminate best practices

Abbreviations: MBA, masters in business administration; MPH, masters in public health; MS, masters of science; PhD, doctor of philosophy.

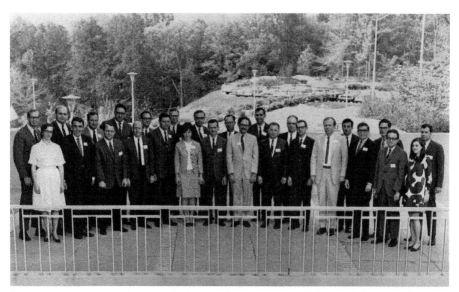

Fig. 2. NIMH career teacher award winners, 1967. Front row (*left to right*): Joan Webb, Norman Levy, Gordon Deckert, Ken Robson, Unidentified, Lenore Terr, Charles Butler, Joel Konel, Unidentified, Unidentified, Braxton McKee, Unidentified, Unidentified, Carol Nadelson. Second Row: Herb Walker, Layton McCurdy, David Dorosin, Samuel Wagonford, Jack Barchas, Martin Harris, John Griffen, Lou Rittlemeyer, Peter Grunberg, Hugh Paul Gabriel, Joe Katsuranis, George Vaillant, Dick Wallace. (*Courtesy of* C. Cooperman Nadelson, MD, Boston, MA.)

career teacher conferences, the first of which took place in Atlanta, Georgia, in 1968 (**Fig. 2**); a second in Palo Alto, California, in 1969; and a third in Charleston, South Carolina, in 1970. With the encouragement of Dr Bernard Bandler, who later oversaw the NIMH training programs, the group formed an organization for psychiatric educators called the Society for Academic Psychiatry, which included career teacher award winners and others. The first Society for Academic Psychiatry annual meeting was held in Boston in 1971, with Dr Larry Silver as inaugural president. The organization renamed itself the AAP—a far more favorable acronym. The AAPs success has been attributed to its fulfilling professional development needs by focusing on teaching techniques and serving as a networking community of like-minded individuals. Today, AAP helps psychiatrists to develop skills and knowledge in teaching, research, and career development and provides members an interactive forum to exchange ideas on teaching techniques, curricula, and problem-solving educational issues, focusing more on process than content.[26]

The evolution of the ADMSEP, described by Dr Fred Sierles,[13] began when a group of East Coast psychiatrists first met in Chicago, Illinois, in 1975. The group focused on issues concerning the NIMH's departmental grants for behavioral science programs and the National Board of Medical Examiners newly initiated part 1 behavioral science section. Medical schools needed psychiatric educators devoted to undergraduate medical education who had broad information and skills to deal with psychiatry's rapidly changing scope, from psychoanalytic theory and efforts to humanize medicine through all the burgeoning new information in psychiatric diagnosis, psychopharmacology and neuroscience. In addition, national concerns regarding the recruitment of medical students into psychiatry predominated in the 1990s. The organization's goals (paraphrased) have included to:

1. Champion excellence in medical student psychiatric education with objectives and professional development of leaders;
2. Facilitate research and innovation in teaching;
3. Collaborate with other psychiatric and medical education organizations to pursue common interests; and
4. Provide support, guidance, and resources to medical students considering psychiatric careers.[27]

The AADPRT, founded in 1970 to further the education and professional development of psychiatry educators and program coordinators, was inspired by Dr Iago Galdston, the first president.[28] Although focusing on primarily education, the AADPRT has also had a political dimension from the beginning, initially related to advancing NIMH funding for psychiatric training. The AADPRT quickly developed relationships with the American Medical Association, APA, American Board of Psychiatry and Neurology (ABPN) and the Residency Review Committee, which continue today. In the late 1990s, advanced psychiatric fellowship directors joined the organization; subsequently, a new training directors symposium and a separate coordinator's symposium were added.

FD related to clinical practice—often called professional development—is directed by many organizations. The ABPN is a nonprofit corporation founded in 1934 following conferences of committees appointed by the APA, the American Neurologic Association, and the then Section on Nervous and Mental Diseases of the American Medical Association. Previously led by Stephen Scheiber and now Larry R. Faulkner, its purpose is to certify psychiatrists' professional achievements after general and subspecialty psychiatric training. Subspecialty organizations, specialized groups (eg, psychopharmacology) and interprofessional fields (eg, neurobiology) contribute to clinical care standards as well. As clinical practice continues to evolve, the APA and ABPN attempt to help clinicians to ensure safe, quality, evidence-based care and to ensure lifelong learning. The Psychiatry Residency Review Committee, a component of the ACGME, has principal responsibility for setting minimal standards and content for adult, child, and adolescent and other psychiatric specialty training programs.

The APA has been centrally involved in promoting psychiatric educators with FD opportunities. Dr Carolyn Robinowitz, who had previously directed medical student education at George Washington University, was recruited by Dr Melvin Sabshin, executive director of the APA, to become the founding director of the APA Office of Education in 1976. At about the same time that NIMH funding for psychiatric education-oriented programs was being terminated, she helped to convene the major national psychiatric education organizations to discuss matters of mutual interest and to coordinate activities by appointing representatives of these organizations to the Council of Education. Consequently, the APA became an organizing vehicle, and conferences such as the Psychiatrist as a Teacher in 1976 encouraged collaboration, sharing of resources and a unified voice. Simultaneously, outreach to AAMC related to the psychiatrist as educator theme focused on medical school curricula and shifting and optimal settings for psychiatric clinical education of medical students. Some of these activities were documented in *Training Psychiatrists for the 90s*.[29] The activities of the APA's current Council on Medical Education and Lifelong Learning continue to serve these coordinating functions in the service of all levels of psychiatric education, including FD.

PSYCHIATRIC ACADEMIC ORGANIZATIONS: PERSPECTIVES AND NARRATIVES FROM SELECTED LEADERS AND PARTICIPANTS
Academic Psychiatry

In 1987, the AADPRT became a founding sponsor of the *Journal of Psychiatric Education* (the title aligned with the AAMC's then extant *Journal of Medical Education*). The founding editor in chief, Dr Zebulon Taintor, had been an AADPRT president. To align with the AAMC education journal's branding shift to *Academic Medicine*, the journal was subsequently renamed *Academic Psychiatry* (*AP*) in 1989. The AAP joined AADPRT in rejuvenating the journal, with Dr Jonathan Borus, emanating from AAP, as editor, and then AADPRT President William Sledge as deputy editor. *AP* focused on attracting and publishing the best articles on psychiatric educational research and programmatic and curricular innovation. Because in most academic settings promotion is tied to one's publishing record, *AP* prioritized the growth of early (usually young) psychiatric educators as writers and reviewers. *AP* developed a policy of providing authors with teaching reviews in which they received, often over several revisions, rapid feedback on ways to improve their manuscript and their writing. The close collaboration between editors and authors contributes to *AP*'s significant ongoing impact on FD.[30]

These missions of *AP* continued under the journal's subsequent editors—Drs Samuel Keith, Paul Mohl, and notably Laura Roberts, who has greatly enhanced its scope, distribution, and readership. *AP*'s official mission is to further knowledge and stimulate evidence-based advances in academic medicine in 6 key domains: education, leadership, finance and administration, career and professional development, ethics and professionalism, and health and well-being. Happily, *AP* is now a major vehicle for sharing educational research and innovation for both psychiatric and nonpsychiatric medical educators.

American Association of Directors of Psychiatric Residency Training
Involvement in AADPRT benefits members in 3 major ways: information dissemination, networking, and leadership development.[12] Through core program events at annual meetings, attendees are regularly updated on new innovations, activities, enacted policies, new regulatory requirements, and emerging proposals of the numerous agencies and governing bodies with which academic psychiatry interacts, most notably the ACGME Residency Review Committee, the ABPN, APA (Office of Education), and the NIMH. Meetings have also been used to train psychiatric educators in conducting nationally required competency examinations in their home programs.

The AADPRT has fostered the development of numerous task forces, essentially special interest groups that bring together faculty with shared interests to collect data, problem solve, craft policy recommendations, model curricula, and often publish their efforts. Innumerable life-long collaborations (and friendships) initiated through these activities have enriched careers and the entire field, particularly with respect to clinician educators.[31] Among others, FD innovations have included development of formal on-site and distance mentorship programs, a train the trainer's manual and workshops, and identification of research literacy as an competency for psychiatric educators. The latter led to development of a series of NIMH-funded premeetings that focus on research methods, statistics, neuroscience, and the nuances of reading and teaching psychiatric research publications, all aimed at psychiatric educators. AADPRT's virtual training office, virtual classroom, and model curricula continue to provide just-in-time resources for psychiatric educators and programs throughout the year. Current efforts include expanding AADPRT's role in FD, with surveys of needs[32] and activities ranging from wellness and resilience to assisting faculty grapple with ACGME milestones, complex health systems, program finances, and a whole host of other challenges.

Narrative by Dr Sandra M. DeJong

My first contact with AADPRT was as a second-year child and adolescent psychiatric fellow at the 2001 Annual Meeting in Seattle, when I was invited to serve as discussant to Tanya Luhrmann's plenary on her recently released book *Of Two Minds*,[33] an anthropologist's look at contemporary psychiatry and its Cartesian split. An earthquake had occurred and Joel Yager, the faculty discussant, was unable to come, and I was left to present solo. I spoke in part about the importance of my training directors' influence on my career and on my thinking: Sheldon Benjamin, my general psychiatry training director, was a neuropsychiatrist; Julia Matthews, Assistant Training Director, a psychoanalyst; and Gene Beresin, my child and adolescent training director, eclectic and all-encompassing. I will always be grateful for the warm reception I received.

Three years later, I returned as a training director myself. I got to know Drs James Lomax, Lisa Mellman, Joan Anzia, Rick Summers, and Adrienne Bentman to name a few. AADPRT, itself, and the mentoring relationships I formed there, have been safe havens in which to discuss all manner of questions, uncertainties, and self-doubts about psychiatry, education, academic development, professional relationships, personal hardships, and more. I always return from AADPRT meetings with gratitude both toward my home institution and for the opportunity to think about my role there from a broader perspective. As Dr Yager describes, "Being a training director can feel like a process of muddling along, albeit with intention." AADPRT mentors provided beacons in that journey along unclear paths.

The AADPRT has also been a wonderful organization for learning. From practical tips on the listserv to inspirational plenaries, like those by psychoanalyst Dr Salman Akhtar or poet Donald Hall, to workshops on everything from using technology for evaluations to structural competence, the AADPRT has provided a forum in which to learn, grow and flourish as a training director. My role as chair of the Presidential Taskforce on Professionalism and the Internet launched my career as an educational scholar, including my first publication in *AP*. I suspect many have had a similar experience.

The theme of the 2018 AADPRT annual meeting was shaping the future of psychiatry. Training directors are shaped at the annual meeting and in turn, shape others as we teach, mentor, and supervise our trainees.

Association for Academic Psychiatry

The AAP played a critical role in my career development as a psychiatry educator and leader. My personal involvement began in late 1975 when Dr Fred Guggenheim invited me to the Northeast Regional meeting of AAP (in a Vermont monastery) and then solidified when he encouraged me to come with him to the March 1976 annual meeting in Denver, Colorado. The warmth and welcome I received from AAP members at that meeting, as well as the impromptu ski trip to Vail with several new colleagues that followed, bonded me to the AAP. Psychiatric education was valued and I could engage with like-minded colleagues with and from whom to learn to be a better educator. Although I have also had the privilege to serve as a long-time residency director, a departmental chair, and as a member of the AADPRT Executive Committee and the APA's Council on Medical Education, the warmth and noncompetitive ambiance of AAP made it my favorite organization. I could discuss problems I was facing in my departmental role, try out new ideas in a safe environment, and develop projects with a network of colleagues from around the country. My investment in the AAP as my primary organization led to my serving as president from 1986 to 1988, and as a department leader I made sure that my best young faculty educators got involved with AAP—and like me, once they went to an AAP annual meeting they were hooked!

The AAP has been the most influential professional organization in my career. I first heard about the AAP from Dr Don Hilty, then AAP President, who encouraged me to go to an annual meeting in Chicago, in 2005, where Dr Joel Yager was the keynote speaker. He introduced himself as, "Hi, my name is Joel, and I am an academic." I was instantly drawn in and leaving the meeting, at the airport bookstore, I found a reference mentioned by him, Malcom Gladwell's *Blink*.[34] I was fascinated by the notion of unconscious bias, researched it, and presented workshops on this topic soon thereafter. Now, it is required reading for leaders in academic medicine.

The secret ingredient of the AAP's culture is mentorship. One doesn't just find mentors at AAP; the entire organization is a living, breathing organism dedicated to mentorship and the advancement of psychiatric education. Everyone is warm and welcoming to first-time attendees and new members. Senior colleagues who you look up to remember your name and are genuinely interested in your life from one year to the other. AAP presidents and residents alike are on first-name basis, an aspect that takes some getting used to and is still baffling to me, after all these years. The feedback from educational consultants after presenting a workshop is meaningful and can lead to lasting changes in your teaching style, particularly when the consultant is Dr Ivan Silver, who helped create the Center for Faculty Development at the University of Toronto!

Another amazing thing, for which I will be forever grateful, was Dr Hilty introducing me to Dr Linda Worley, who took on the AAP presidency reins at the 2005 Annual Meeting. Ever since, Linda has been a beloved mentor and friend who, despite being incredibly busy in her highly successful career, still finds time for long walks with me during the annual meeting, to help me decipher the challenges of midcareer faculty life. Not surprisingly, meeting her and so many others at the AAP, informed my work at UC Davis. We founded an FD group called the Society for Women in Academic Psychiatry in the Department, which is still active.[35] This work opened many doors and brought several leadership opportunities, culminating in a position of Associate Dean for Student Wellness at UC Davis.

The AAP offers many opportunities for FD and collaboration. Chief among these is the Master Educator program, a longitudinal series of workshops offered at the annual meeting, centered on adult learning theory, new teaching methods, program evaluation, educational scholarship, and other topics.[36]

Association of Directors of Medical Student Education in Psychiatry

Twenty-two years ago, I became a psychiatry clerkship director. A perk of the job was a trip to the annual meeting of ADMSEP. I quickly discovered that this small group of friendly like-minded educators would become my professional family. Every year we meet, and like family we came to know each other and engage in holiday-like rituals of hearty celebration and vigorous debate about the issues surrounding medical student education. Initially we were less than 100 in number, but new clerkship directors were welcomed into the fold with enthusiasm and shared in the closeness and camaraderie.

More important, from a professional perspective, I discovered a treasure trove of wisdom and opportunity for collaboration and mentorship. Members discovered in one another the opportunity to network not only for support but also for scholarship and advancement. Through the ADMSEP, my colleagues developed textbooks, standardized clerkship objectives, and generated position statements. I learned that these colleagues were an indispensable resource for the knowledge and skills of how to conduct research and nurture collaborative scholarly relationships. One of my earliest educational research publications was coauthored by the ADMSEP pioneer Dr Fred Sierles, who taught me about the challenges of survey research. Soon afterward, 3 other ADMSEP colleagues and I engaged in my first significant educational research project. That project led to many more and, reflecting back, I realize that a great deal of my professional work including collaborative research, presentations, and publications came about through my interactions with these colleagues.

As important, through ADMSEP I have developed lifelong friendships. Six years ago I moved away from being a clerkship director, becoming an assistant then an associate dean. Nevertheless, I have not yet missed a meeting, still enjoying the opportunity to mentor the next generation of medical student educators. ADMSEP is no longer an organization just for clerkship directors, in that it now welcomes all psychiatric medical student educators. As such it has grown substantially over the years and now includes programs for coordinators, development for educational scholars, and expanded opportunities for grants, awards, and other recognition. About 85% of all medical schools in the United States have faculty membership and ADMSEP now has a list serve, newsletter, and even a LinkedIn group. Recently, ADMSEP members have developed libraries of eModules, innovative curricula, and cutting edge learning objects on the website and in collaboration with the AAMC. There are innumerable opportunities for networking and collaboration, with multiple committees, task forces, and special interest groups. Nevertheless the organization remains a friendly environment where new members are welcomed and mentorship is celebrated.

American College of Psychiatrists
The American College of Psychiatrists comprises more than 750 psychiatrists who have demonstrated excellence in the field of psychiatry and achieved national recognition in clinical practice, research, academic leadership, or teaching. It specifically oversees the Psychiatry Residency In Training Examination, an educational resource for psychiatric residents and training programs, and the Improvement in Medical Practice Examination, a comprehensive online examination allowing clinicians to assess their knowledge and skills throughout their careers. It is also used to prepare psychiatrists for ABPN certification and maintenance of certification and fulfill the ABPN's self-assessment and lifelong learning maintenance of certification requirement.

American Psychiatric Press Publishing
The American Psychiatric Press Publishing is the world's premier publisher of books, journals, and multimedia on psychiatry, mental health, and behavioral science. As a division of the APA, its purposes are to distribute publications of the APA and to publish books independent of the policies and procedures of the APA. It was founded in 1981 and Drs Shervert Frazier, Robert E. Hales, and Carol C. Nadelson have served as past editors in chief. It is now overseen by current Editors-in-Chief Dr Laura Roberts and John McDuffie.

DISCUSSION

From the start, the NIMH and the several national psychiatric organizations have provided good teaching and mentoring options. At the same time, informal mentoring remains crucial for faculty satisfaction, self-efficacy, socialization,[37] and retention,[38] partly to reduce stress and isolation and to set realistic expectations. Regardless of available resources or limitations in various local departmental and institutional settings, faculty have to take initiative, collaborate with others and seize opportunities.

Because the scope of FD is broad across clinical, educational, research and administrative areas, productivity and socialization can be facilitated via multifaceted mentoring programs for early career faculty, structured annual faculty reviews and project-based FD.[22,39,40]

Creating successful cultures for FD calls for improvement in several areas including better day-to-day practice of wellness, specifically prevention of bad outcomes such as burnout and suicide,[41] better definitions of academic success, and attention to concepts of academic "", keys for aligning personal and organizational values.[42] Finally, recruiting, developing, and supporting a more diverse faculty, better representing the population at large, is also mandatory in light of the disadvantages and barriers that so many face in obtaining health care.[43,44]

As psychiatry moves forward as a profession, contributions from individuals, departments, institutions, and national organizations will be critical. Organizational activities such as informal apprenticeships, mentoring, and longitudinal team-based guided learning will continue to be central elements in ensuring the competent development of future faculty. Implementing robust, continually evolving and evaluated FD processes will ensure high-quality care, meet professional standards, and encourage the innovation necessary for successfully negotiating the rapidly changing practices of psychiatry. Effective process and structure (eg, well-mentored MD/PhD and K award programs for research)[45] for FD is paramount to helping our clinical, educational and research missions.

ACKNOWLEDGMENTS

The authors would like to acknowledge the following individuals for their contributions to this article: Dr Layton McCurdy, Dean Emeritus and Professor of Psychiatry and Behavioral Sciences at the Medical University of South Carolina, Charleston, South Carolina; former President, American Board of Psychiatry and Neurology; and former President, American College of Psychiatrists. Dr Carolyn B. Robinowitz, Founding Director, American Psychiatric Office of Education; former Dean, Georgetown School of Medicine; former President, American Board of Psychiatry and Neurology; former President of the Council of Medical Specialty Societies. Dr Carol C. Nadelson, Brigham and Women's Hospital; former President, American Psychiatric Association; second Editor-In-Chief of American Psychiatric Press Publishing; Fellow, American Academy of Arts and Sciences.

REFERENCES

1. Kirch DG. The role of academic psychiatry in the transformation of health care. Acad Psychiatry 2011;35(2):73–5.
2. Hilty DM, Srinivasan M, Xiong G, et al. Lessons from psychiatry and psychiatric education for medical learners and teachers. Int Rev Psychiatry 2013;25:329–37.
3. Yager J. Personal reflections on a life of learning and teaching psychiatry. Int Rev Psychiatry 2013;25(3):357–63.
4. Pratt DD. Five perspectives on teaching in adult and higher education. Malabar (FL): Krieger Publishing; 1998.
5. Corrice A, Fox S, Bunton S, Association of American Medical Colleges. Retention of full-time clinical MD faculty at US medical schools, February 2011, AAMC Analysis in Brief. Available at: https://www.aamc.org/download/175974/data/aibvol11_no2.pdf. Accessed December 27, 2018.
6. Weerasekera P. Psychiatric organizations: influencing professional development. Acad Psychiatry 2007;31(2):89–90.

7. Bland CJ, Schmitz CC, Stritter FT, et al. Successful faculty in academic medicine: essential skills and how to acquire them. New York: Springer; 1990.

8. Steinert Y, Naismith L, Mann K. Faculty development initiatives designed to promote leadership in medical education. A BEME systematic review: BEME Guide No. 19. Med Teach 2012;34(6):483–503.

9. Steinert YG. Faculty development in the health professions. (Netherlands): Springer; 2014. p. 3–25.

10. Liu H, Hilty DM. Defining professional development in psychiatry, medicine and allied fields. P Clin N Amer, in press.

11. Armstrong EG, Mackey M, Spear SJ. Medical education as a process management problem. Acad Med 2004;79(8):721–8.

12. Mellman LA. Cultivating careers in the American Association of Directors of Psychiatric Residency Training. Acad Psychiatry 2007;31(2):101–2.

13. Sierles FS. The Association of Directors of Medical Student Education in Psychiatry. Acad Psychiatry 2007;31(2):107–9.

14. Baron DA. How the AACDP helped me professionally and personally. Acad Psychiatry 2007;31(2):99–100.

15. Harden RM, Crosby JR, Davis MH. AMEE guide no. 14: outcome-based education: part 1—An introduction to outcome-based education. Med Teach 1999;21: 7–14. Available at: http://www.deu.edu.tr/UploadedFiles/Birimler/ 16781/R%20M %20HARDEN%20(Outcome%20based%20education)%20MAKALE.pdf. Accessed December 27, 2018.

16. Steinert Y, Mann K, Anderson B, et al. A systematic review of faculty development initiatives designed to enhance teaching effectiveness: a 10-year update: BEME Guide No. 40. Med Teach 2016;38(8):769–86.

17. Roberts LW, Hilty DM. Handbook of career development in academic psychiatry and behavioral sciences. 2nd edition. American Psychiatric Press Publishing; 2017.

18. Hales RE, Shahrokh NC, Servis M. A progress report on a department of psychiatry faculty practice plan designed to reward educational and research productivity. Acad Psychiatry 2009;33(3):248–51.

19. Teshima J, Seritan A, Myint MT, et al. Developmental approaches to Faculty development. P Clin N Amer, in press.

20. Srinivasan M, Li ST, Meyers FJ, et al. Teaching as a competency for medical educators: competencies for medical educators. Acad Med 2011;86(10):1211–20.

21. Hilty DM, Crawford A, Teshima J, et al. A framework for telepsychiatric training and e-health: competency-based education, evaluation and implications. Int Rev Psychiatry 2015;27(6):569–92.

22. Mennin S, Kalishman S, Eklund M, et al. Project-based faculty development by international health professions educators: practical strategies. Med Teach 2013;35:e971–7.

23. Davis D, Evans M, Jadad A, et al. The case for knowledge translation: shortening the journey from evidence to effect. BMJ 2003;327(7405):33–5.

24. O'Sullivan PS, Irby DM. Reframing research on faculty development. Acad Med 2011;86(4):421–8.

25. Arnhoff FN, Shriver BM, VanMatre RM. Subsequent career activities of National Institute of Mental Health trainees in psychiatry. J Med Educ 1967;42(9):855–62.

26. Association for Academic Psychiatry. 2018. Available at: https://www. academicpsychiatry.org. Accessed December 27, 2018.

27. Association of Directors of Medical Student Education in Psychiatry. 2018. Available at: http://www.admsep.org. Accessed December 27, 2018.

28. American Association of Directors of Psychiatry Residency Training. 2018. Available at: https://www.aadprt.org. Accessed December 27, 2018.

29. Nadelson CC, Robinowitz CB. Training psychiatrists for the '90s: issues and recommendations (issues in psychiatry). Washington, DC: American Psychiatric Publishing, Incorporated; 1987.

30. Borus JF. Editors and authors: two halves of a whole. Acad Psychiatry 2014;38(2): 224–5.

31. Yager J, Ritvo A, Wolfe JH, et al. A survival guide to low-resource peer-reviewed creative scholarship for aspiring clinician-educators. Acad Psychiatry 2018. https://doi.org/10.1007/s40596-018-0969-4.

32. De Golia SG, Cagande CC, Ahn MS, et al. Faculty development for teaching faculty in psychiatry: where we are and what we need. Acad Psychiatry 2018. https://doi.org/10.1007/s40596-018-0916-4.

33. Luhrmann T. Of two minds: an anthropologist looks at American psychiatry. New York: Random House; 2000.

34. Gladwell M. Blink: the power of thinking without thinking. New York: Little, Brown and Company; 2005.

35. Seritan AL, Bhangoo R, Garma S, et al. Society for women in academic psychiatry: a peer mentoring approach. Acad Psychiatry 2007;31(5):363–6.

36. Blitzstein S, Seritan A, Sockalingham S, et al. From industry to generativity: the first twelve years of the Association for Academic Psychiatry Master Educator Program. Acad Psychiatry 2016;40(4):576–83.

37. Shollen SL, Bland CJ, Center BA, et al. Relating mentor type and mentoring behaviors to academic medicine faculty satisfaction and productivity at one medical school. Acad Med 2014;89(9):1267–75.

38. Allen TD, Eby LT. Factors related to mentor reports of mentoring functions provided: gender and relational characteristics. Sex Roles 2004;50:129–39.

39. Chen MM, Sandborg CI, Hudgins L, et al. A multifaceted mentoring program for junior faculty in academic pediatrics. Teach Learn Med 2016;28(3):320–8.

40. Robboy SJ, McLendon R. Structured annual faculty review program accelerates professional development and promotion: long-term experience of the Duke University Medical Center's pathology department. Acad Pathol 2017;4. 2374289516689471.

41. Corbett BA, Marla V, Nanda N, et al. Taking care of yourself. In: Roberts LW, Hilty DM, editors. Handbook of career development in academic psychiatry and behavioral sciences. 2nd edition. Washington, DC: American Psychiatric Press Publishing; 2017. p. 373–84.

42. Leslie K. Faculty development for academic and career development. In: Steinert YG, editor. Faculty development in the health professions. (Netherlands): Springer; 2014. p. 97–118.

43. Rodriguez JE, Campbell KM, Fogarty JP, et al. Underrepresented minority faculty in academic medicine: a systematic review of URM faculty development. Fam Med 2014;46(2):100–4.

44. Nivet MA. A Diversity 3.0 update: are we moving the needle enough? Acad Med 2015;90(12):1591–3.

45. Marsh JD, Todd RF 3rd. Training and sustaining physician scientists: what is success? Am J Med 2015;128(4):431–6.

Developmental Approaches to Faculty Development

John Teshima, BSc, MEd, MD, FRCPC[a],*, Alastair J.S. McKean, MD[b],
Myo Thwin Myint, MD[c], Shadi Aminololama-Shakeri, MD[d], Shashank V. Joshi, MD[e],
Andreea L. Seritan, MD[f], Donald M. Hilty, MD, MBA[g]

KEYWORDS

- Faculty development • Early career • Mid-career • Late career
- Developmental stages

KEY POINTS

- An academic career goes through developmental stages, and faculty have different needs as they progress through these different stages.
- Early-career faculty need mentorship and orientation programs to help develop their clinical and academic identities.
- Mid-career faculty benefit from programs that provide new skills and leadership training to help with role transitions and generativity.
- Advanced-career faculty benefit from mentorship as they focus on integration, contributing, and changes in roles and power.

INTRODUCTION

Any longitudinal human endeavor involving the progression from novice to expert can be viewed from a developmental perspective. The career of an academic psychiatrist is no exception. Over a career, an academic psychiatrist develops greater and

Disclosure: The authors have nothing to disclose.
[a] Department of Psychiatry, University of Toronto, Sunnybrook Health Sciences Centre, 2075 Bayview Avenue, Room FG-62, Toronto, Ontario M4N 3M5, Canada; [b] Department of Psychiatry and Psychology, Mayo Clinic, 200 First Street Southwest, Rochester, MN 55905, USA; [c] Department of Psychiatry and Behavioral Sciences, and Pediatrics, Tulane University, 1430 Tulane Avenue, #8055, New Orleans, LA 70112, USA; [d] Department of Radiology, University of California Davis, 4860 Y Street, Suite 3100, Sacramento, CA 95817, USA; [e] Division of Child and Adolescent Psychiatry, Stanford University School of Medicine, 401 Quarry Road, Room 1119, Stanford, CA 94305-5719, USA; [f] Department of Psychiatry, University of California, San Francisco, UCSF Weill Institute for Neurosciences, 401 Parnassus Avenue, Box 0984-APC, San Francisco, CA 94143, USA; [g] Department of Psychiatry and Behavioral Sciences, Mental Health, Northern California Veterans Administration Health Care System, University of California Davis, 10535 Hospital Way, Mather, CA 95655, USA
* Corresponding author.
E-mail address: john.teshima@utoronto.ca

Psychiatr Clin N Am 42 (2019) 375–387
https://doi.org/10.1016/j.psc.2019.05.008
0193-953X/19/© 2019 Elsevier Inc. All rights reserved.

increasingly sophisticated knowledge and skills in all of their professional activities: clinical care, academic activities (eg, research, teaching, mentorship, and quality improvement), leadership, and administration. However, development over a career is not just about gaining knowledge and skills. Goals and priorities can change over time; attitudes and perspectives can shift. Many of these changes can be influenced by events and processes occurring outside of the career, including family life, personal health and the health of others, financial situations, and other factors.

Theories of adult development and identity development can be mapped on to career stages and trajectories. Various authors have explored and elaborated on Erik Erikson's theory of psychosocial development as applied to careers.[1,2] Erikson's stage 5 (Identity vs Role Confusion) can be connected to the challenges at the beginning of a career, when a person is trying to establish a professional identity, and failure to do so can lead to a crisis of identity in general. Concerns of Generativity versus Stagnation (Erikson's stage 7) can become increasingly prominent in mid-career and Ego Integrity versus Despair (stage 8) can dominate the later years. These authors also note that a career goes through many periods of transition. Thus, an academic career can be also seen as progressing through what James Marcia describes as "identity moratorium," in which individuals are in crisis and exploring options and then "identity achievement," in which individuals have made choices and are pursuing goals consistent with their newly established identities.[3]

Bourgeois and Servis more recently applied George Vaillant's adult development framework, itself based on Eriksonian stages, to the career of an academic psychiatrist.[4] They identified that the first stage "Identity" begins in medical school and early residency, when an individual begins developing clinical skills. The stage of "Intimacy" occurs primarily in residency, when there is the solidification of collegial relationship and the development of trust and reliance in colleagues. "Career Consolidation" spans late residency into junior faculty years, when there is both further strengthening of clinical expertise and the initial commitment to a career pathway. "Generativity" covers the junior faculty to mid-career faculty, when there is more emphasis on teaching and mentoring trainees and more junior colleagues. "Keeper of the Meaning" is the stage in which more senior faculty are in positions of leadership and establishing future directions. Lastly, "Integrity" applies to retiring faculty, who have a sense of satisfaction of their achievements and are still providing sage advice to leadership.

Given these understandings of academic faculty having different goals, needs, skills, and tasks at different career stages, it only makes sense to provide different faculty development programs and initiatives for the different career stages.[5,6] However, defining career stages is not so simple and clear cut.[7] Although academic careers are often defined by academic rank, there are faculty who are rapidly promoted based on their academic productivity, but in many other ways still have the needs of more junior faculty. There are also many seasoned faculty who are incredibly generative and provide leadership, and yet for various reasons have stalled at the Assistant Professor level. It is also not clear that all domains of an academic career (clinical, research, education, leadership, and so forth) develop in lockstep with each other.

It is also important to recognize that some issues affect faculty across all career stages. Academic medicine is in the process of change in many areas:

1. Health care reforms are changing medical practice and health care delivery systems
2. Decreased funding for academic activity is resulting in shifting strategies to address the financial shortfalls
3. Educational innovations are changing where and how learners are being trained[8]

Faculty development is needed to help all faculty adapt to these new challenges.

Notwithstanding these complexities, this article reviews the faculty development literature relevant to each career stage (early, mid, and advanced), and make recommendations about faculty development approaches (content, processes) for each stage.

EARLY CAREER

> In his residency, Dr. M established a reputation for excellence in his clinical skills, work ethic, research efforts, and educational initiatives. On completion of his fellowship training, he was quickly recruited by the chair. In the year following, Dr. M observed that he was becoming increasingly frustrated in his role. He found the transition to junior faculty more challenging than he expected. He was confused by the departmental committees and bureaucracy, and was challenged in balancing a multitude of tasks. Dr. M had also struggled to find a suitable mentor and also to find the time to meet. Adding to these concerns was departmental attrition, with 2 other junior psychiatrists recently leaving for private practice. The redistribution of their workload, combined with more senior colleagues passing on administrative duties and responsibilities, meant that the things he valued—education and research—were shrinking from his calendar at an alarming rate. Dr. M had less time available for his young children and partner, as his evenings and weekends became progressively devoted to the research and educational activities that had been pushed out of his regular schedule. Maybe his recently departed junior colleagues had made the right decision? Perhaps, he thought, he should be looking at other options too.
>
> What can Dr. M's department and school do to help him succeed at this stage?

An early-career psychiatrist faces developmental challenges that map onto Erickson's fifth stage of development—Identity vs Role Confusion.[4] They are trying to establish their identity and expertise in their clinical area and in their area of academic focus.[7] Early-stage careers in academic medicine are particularly vulnerable to attrition. Approximately 10% of physicians enter into academic careers, with roughly a third of these physicians leaving after 3 years, and half departing academia within a decade of starting.[9] There are many factors contributing to this erosion. Some individuals will recognize that an academic career does not suit their talents, ambitions, or life outside of work, and depart to new endeavors. Others may be suited to these paths but choose not to persist in them, possibly related to a poor goodness-of-fit between physician and the ethos of his or her institution. Some women specifically choose to leave owing to personal and family reasons.[10] But, in many cases, this departure from academia may be related to inadequate support and faculty development that diminish the prospect of advancement.[11–13]

Given the financial and administrative costs of losing faculty, there is pressure on academic centers to ensure retention and development.[14] The transitional years following completion of training into a nascent faculty role are a vulnerable time requiring support and nurturing in order for the junior academician to take root in his or her new role. How should psychiatry departments grow and develop the early careers of psychiatrists in this environment? How do junior faculty members access the necessary support to sustain and flourish in an academic psychiatry career? Given the diverse needs and backgrounds of incoming early-career psychiatrists, there is no singular approach to fostering development. Early-career growth may require a plurality of approaches depending on the needs of the clinician and the capacities of the department in which they practice.

The longstanding mainstay of early-career development has been the traditional mentor-mentee dyad. This model relies on a mentor, who with experience, skill, and knowledge guides and supports a mentee as they grow into a similar role. This model can occur informally, with the relationship occurring through mutual interest or compatibility, or, more formally, with departments arranging or stipulating the relationship.[15] Although this dyad is the model that most people think of when considering mentorship, it has been limited in that not all junior faculty members have access to individual mentors.[16] In addition, identifying time to build this relationship and finding a mentor who is a good fit can be challenging. It is also recognized that singular connections, regardless of strength, may prove too limited to the nascent academic.

Peer-mentoring groups provide an alternative to this traditional dyad, whereby early-career clinicians meet together to share knowledge, skills, and support with one another. This model has been used in lieu of, or in conjunction with, dyadic mentorship models of faculty development, and has been noted to produce greater productivity, career satisfaction, and collaboration.[17–19] It is also likely that these collaborations can strengthen departments holistically because better connections and professional relationships are formed between junior faculty members.

Some institutions have implemented curricula and formal programs to provide foundational information to junior faculty and to orient them to the institutional culture. These have included seminars,[20] a week-long core curriculum course,[21] and longitudinal programs coupled with mentoring processes.[14,22] Programs such as these recognize the discrepancy between the knowledge and skills new faculty arrive with and what they need to be successful. Comprehensive curricula can help with identifying a mentor, applying for grants, writing papers, cultivating work-life balance, and networking.

Finally, an essential component of early-career development is networking with other psychiatrists. Gaining multiple perspectives from different individuals across institutions can enrich and advance early careers.[23] Professional organizations offer access to networking events at annual meetings and through membership. In addition, social media can play an important role in connecting people with a wider assortment of mentors through Facebook, LinkedIn, or even Twitter.[24] There is increasing recognition that multiple mentors are needed for success and developing particular skills in certain areas.[23] The business literature suggests that successfully creating a network of mentors is a positive predictor of career development and creates a strength and depth of support that a smaller, more traditional mentorship model cannot offer.[23,25,26]

Ultimately, new faculty require the support of many through a variety of different modalities and settings to be successful. Mentorship dyads, peer-mentoring groups, and faculty development curricula are not always available. Effective networking, however, offers the potential to bridge deficiencies that junior faculty members may face at their institution.

MID-CAREER

Dr. A is an academic psychiatrist who was recently promoted to associate professor. At the same time, she became the Child and Adolescent Psychiatry division chief and was asked to run the residency scholarship curriculum, which included a series of lectures and small groups for first- through fourth-year residents, culminating in a 2-day symposium at which all residents presented their scholarly projects. In addition to her departmental roles, Dr. A had been working with her national professional organization for 5 years, and was now running the education committee and working on several projects. Dr. A had also been sponsored by a more senior woman at her medical school and was next in line to chair the clinical curriculum committee, a stepping stone to an associate dean for curriculum position. Dr. A, already a busy clinician and mother of 2 teenage children, found herself inundated with emails and meetings related to these additional responsibilities. She started waking up 2 hours earlier and going to bed later, and stopped exercising. After 3 months, Dr. A felt exhausted, ineffective, irritable, and emotionally unavailable to her family. Her research projects had fallen by the wayside and she felt chronically behind. She fantasized about leaving academia, even though she loved her work, in particular being with her patients and trainees.

What can Dr. A's department and school do to help her succeed at this stage?

This case vignette illustrates the complexities of roles that many academic physicians encounter in mid-career years. As noted previously, academic institutions and professional organizations invest in early-career faculty development programs. However, once faculty reach the associate professor stage, support becomes scarce and faculty development programs are less robust.[27–30]

The mid-career stage aligns with Erikson's adult development stages of Career Consolidation and Generativity, as described above.[4] At this juncture, physicians withstand multiple pressures, as in the vignette above, and undergo complex changes determined both by their intrinsic motivations and the need to adapt to external factors. Some will seek to add depth to areas they are already proficient in, such as improving their teaching skills or developing a new focus of clinical expertise, whereas others may venture into new fields and pursue additional degrees in administration, health professions education, public health, or other sciences.[31,32] This continuous drive for growth and lifelong learning is typical of academic physicians and other highly generative professions.[4,31] Role transitions uncover the need for optimal succession planning. Mid-career physicians who have successfully mentored and sponsored junior colleagues will find this stage more rewarding and will more aptly negotiate role changes.[33]

On a personal level, mid-career physicians may have young families and/or aging parents. Life demands, in addition to work stressors, can contribute to increased stress and even burnout.[34,35] The "off-ramp" phenomenon, which refers to highly qualified individuals who take time off for family reasons, has been described particularly for women.[36] However, it is more difficult to reenter academic careers after temporary departures. Even though many academic institutions have family-friendly and "stop the clock" policies, women and men who take advantage of such policies may feel penalized by having to explain gaps in their work histories, reentering at lower ranks than expected, or not being eligible for extramural funding owing to lower recent output of peer-reviewed publications. Moreover, some mid-career faculty (especially women) may leave academia altogether and join practices that allow more flexibility to accommodate family needs.[10] Institutions are encouraged to develop programs that support mid-career physicians and help them cultivate satisfaction and avoid burnout.[35]

Most reported interventions designed for mid-career faculty are in the category of faculty development programs, many of which have been put in place to meet the needs of women and/or underrepresented minority faculty in overcoming obstacles to career progression.[10,19,37] Specifically, interventions designed to help reduce gender and racial bias have been shown to increase recruitment and promotion of more diverse faculty, and change the institutional culture in ways that can promote the career advancement of women in medicine, science, and engineering.[38,39] Although there is inter-institutional variability, most longitudinal programs contain common elements such as: mentorship, leadership training, and new skills development.[19,37,38] With regard to measuring the effectiveness of such interventions, the

Table 1
Examples of national faculty development programs

Program	Target Faculty Group
Early career	
USA	
AAMC Minority Faculty Leadership Development Seminar: https://www.aamc.org/members/leadership/catalog/323116/minorityfacultyleadership developmentseminar.html	URM (assistant professor)
AAMC Early Career Women Faculty Leadership Development Seminar: https://www.aamc.org/members/leadership/catalog/323134/earlycareerwomenfacultyleadership developmentseminar.html	Women (assistant professor)
Harvard Macy Institute program for Educators in Health Professions: https://www.harvardmacy.org/index.php/hmi-courses/educators	Faculty in educational leadership roles
Mid-career	
Canada	
Canadian Association for Medical Education Canadian Leadership Institute for Medical Education (CLIME): https://www.came-acem.ca/professional-development/clime-iclem/	All faculty in educational leadership roles
CMA Physician Leadership Institute: https://joulecma.ca/learn	All faculty
USA	
AAMC Mid-Career Minority Faculty Leadership Development Seminar: https://www.aamc.org/members/leadership/catalog/452848/mid-careerminorityfaculty leadershipseminar.html	URM (associate professor)
AAMC Mid-Career Women Faculty Leadership Development Seminar: https://www.aamc.org/members/leadership/catalog/323118/mid-careerwomenfacultyleadership developmentseminar.html	Women (associate professor)
American College of Physicians Leadership Academy: https://www.acponline.org/meetings-courses/acp-courses-recordings/acp-leadership-academy	All faculty
Career Advancement & Leadership Skills for Women in Healthcare: https://womens leadership.hmscme.com	Women
Executive Leadership in Academic Medicine (ELAM): https://drexel.edu/medicine/academics/womens-health-and-leadership/elam/	Women (associate professor, at least 2 y at rank)
National Center for Faculty Development and Diversity: https://www.facultydiversity.org/mid-career	All faculty (URM and women in particular)

(continued on next page)

	Target Faculty
Program	**Group**
Late Career	
USA	
AAMC Organizational Leadership in Academic Medicine for New Associate Deans and Department Chairs: https://www.aamc.org/members/leadership/catalog/323132/organization alleadershipinacademicmedicine.html	Associate deans and department chairs (within first 3 y in their roles)
Harvard Macy Institute Leading Innovations in Healthcare and Education https://www.harvardmacy.org/index.php/hmi-courses/leaders	Faculty in AHC leadership roles

Table 1
(continued)

Abbreviations: AAMC, Association of American Medical Colleges; AHC, academic health center; CMA, Canadian Medical Association; URM, underrepresented minorities in medicine.

literature is dominated by qualitative research (participant perception), with few studies measuring the impact on institutional culture, faculty retention, or trainee or patient satisfaction. The educational intervention on addressing gender bias developed at the University of Wisconsin-Madison was a cluster randomized controlled trial.[38]

Academic institutions can also sponsor mid-career faculty to attend national professional development programs. **Table 1** presents examples of such programs. The Executive Leadership in Academic Medicine program offers leadership training for women in academic medicine relying on networking and mentoring strategies, and has been reported to have a positive impact in advancing female faculty's careers.[40,41] The Association of American Medical Colleges Group on Faculty Affairs organizes conferences, mentoring circles, and other development opportunities for all career stages. Another useful resource is the mid-career section of the National Center for Faculty Development and Diversity.

ADVANCED CAREER

> *Dr. Z is a 59-year-old female psychiatrist, in a committed partnership with 2 children, who has worked at an academic center for 26 years. Her areas of interest include clinical care in mood disorders, women's health, and underserved populations. Her time includes 70% clinical care, 20% funded clinical research, and 10% as medical director. She enjoys this work and is considering less clinical care, more time with clinical research, and is also being courted for an associate dean position for faculty development. She mentioned her options to a colleague at a national meeting, stating that the psychiatry chair probably preferred her to stay in the department. She also said that she did not currently have a mentor to discuss options. Instead she was doing a lot to mentor others in psychiatry, particularly other women and was seen as a role model. She was unsure about what next steps to take.*
>
> *What can Dr. Z.'s department and school do to help her succeed at this stage?*

There does not seem to be a decline in competence or productivity as faculty age, but there is often a shift in their priorities and values.[42] Many assume that experienced faculty will know what to do, how to do it, and when to do it. But self-assessment, reflection, and informal processes are no guarantee for clarity, adjusting to change, and dealing with academic stress. The advanced-career stage has good challenges, including a variety of options, choices, and directions (including retirement). It also has difficult challenges, including shifts in identity, loss of roles, and diminished power and authority. A lack of clear goals/expectations, preparation, peer and institutional support, and balance may result in dissatisfaction or feeling undervalued. Personal-professional balance is key, particular with aging, losses, and matters involving extended family and health.

Key roles for advanced-career faculty include mentoring, networking for faculty or departments, career advancement, and/or leading a significant charge for the institution. In this regard, longitudinal approaches are needed for advanced-career faculty to be productive and serve as role models, particularly for generations with potentially different values and who are key participants in institutional change across professions and health systems. A reappraisal of clinical, research, scholarship, and administrative endeavors is also suggested, as the advanced-career stage is an opportunity for sustained and new growth. Advanced-career strengths (eg, master teacher, research design specialist, and national leader) may be overlooked, but, if used, these may contribute to a sense of community and help prevent burnout and attrition.[30] Many realize that leadership does not need a title,[43] as there is benefit from leading or contributing to programs, services, sites, divisions, and other enterprises overall.

Advanced-career faculty have played instrumental roles as mentors over many decades and at many levels. Mentorship can be divided into career-related (formal) and psychosocial (informal) categories.[44] Formal advice helps with advancement (eg, sponsorship, exposure, visibility, coaching, protection, and challenging assignments). Informal advice enhances interpersonal function and ideally promotes the mentee's sense of competence, self-efficacy, and development (eg, role modeling, friendship, counseling, acceptance, and confirmation of professional self).

Mentors still need their own mentoring. They need an exchange of knowledge and shared learning about career development strategies to address common challenges relating to negotiation of late career and retirement plans. However, advanced-career faculty may have difficulty accessing their own mentors. The shift to distance mentoring based on technology (eg, teleconferencing) may result in regional and national mentoring,[45] including for researchers.[46] As workforce, policies, and programs advance for diversity and inclusion, customized distance mentoring may increase.[47]

Advanced-career faculty can also seek out mentorship through groups. Medicine is moving from one-on-one to groups and from cross-sectional trainings to team- and project-based longitudinal models. In particular, team-, peer-, and interdisciplinary-based projects are becoming more common,[48] and these relationships increase socialization, reduce isolation, and promote shared goals. These faculty development "interventions" also change attitudes toward organizations, provide skills and knowledge, and adjust leadership behaviors in faculty. Workplace-based projects may help the institution attract more resources (eg, faculty and staff knowledge and skills), budgets can be repurposed, and faculty/staff time are rededicated to new projects.

Although not unique to advanced-career faculty, themes of identity, a sense of belonging, and integration (called by many "balance") becomes more important within professional roles and between professional-personal roles.[49] From a process point-of-view, decisions may be framed in terms of individual and professional identity self-definitions, which are constructed over time through the complex interplay of affective, cognitive, and sociocultural factors.[50] Psychological and/or material reinforcements play a role, and, typically, academic faculty often continue to work long-term, owing to reinforcement from more responsibility over patient outcomes, advancement of research, and the education of future generations of physicians. Advanced-career faculty often reflect often about belonging to a professional community, continuity planning, self-efficacy (current competence, overall impact), and aging. Thus, having a community of peer mentors (colleagues who may or may not be older, but who have preceded the faculty member in thriving in the advanced-career stage), becomes very important.

In addition, because many advanced-career faculty are still very active in clinical care, research, and teaching, they will require faculty development related to all of the current changes that are affecting these domains. Advanced-career faculty will need to gain new knowledge and skills related to changes in clinical service delivery, financial and funding models, and curricular innovations if they are to remain effective and vital in their academic roles. They may require particular attention and support, given that some of these changes may represent paradigm shifts, not just updates and modifications.

DISCUSSION

Because faculty have different needs at different career stages, at very least the content of faculty development initiatives should be different at the different career stages. As we have noted above, early-career faculty need to be oriented to their institutional culture. They also need the knowledge and skills required to be successful in launching their clinical and academic careers. Mid-career faculty, having successfully navigated these first steps, are often moving into new endeavors and leadership roles and thus require new knowledge and skills in the areas that will support these transitions. Advanced-career faculty are starting to transition out of their major leadership roles and also have one eye toward retirement in the future. They are also looking to leave a legacy of impact. They need support and guidance in navigating these steps.

Faculty development approaches can be described on continua from informal to formal and from individual to group-based.[30] Formal, group-based programs are particular suitable when there is extensive content that needs to be delivered efficiently to faculty who all have needs in common, such as early-career faculty who need foundational knowledge and skills for their academic careers. Several examples of these types of programs are noted above.[14,21,22] Formal, group-based programs are also suitable for specialized areas of expertise that some faculty may choose to pursue in mid-career or for specific subgroups of faculty who may need particular support at the mid-career stage.

Although there is an increasing number of faculty development programs being offered through specific faculty development offices, the responsibility for these offerings is also distributed among various other university and medical school offices/departments.[51] Faculty affairs offices, in particular, are the predominant provider of many faculty development programs for all career stages. Offices for specific subgroups of faculty (eg, women and minorities) also provide several programs.

Mentorship is critical across all the career stages (**Table 2**). It is a form of intervention that can be individual and informal, as in the traditional dyadic format, or group-based and formal, as in the peer-mentoring format.[17–19] Mentorship can have value for faculty across all career stages. The dyadic and peer formats can be complementary. However, finding appropriate senior mentors at the advanced-career stage can be challenging, with such potential mentors retired or less accessible. Thus the peer-mentoring format may be even more relevant to advanced-career faculty, who can

Table 2
Mentorship needs and roles across the career stages

	Early	Mid	Advanced
Needs	Developing professional identity	Consolidating professional identity	Transitioning out of leadership
	Clinical expertise	Career transitions	Redefining identity
	Academic career development	Leadership	Preparing for retirement
	Wellness	Wellness	Wellness
Formats	Traditional dyadic	Traditional dyadic	Peer primarily, individual or group
	Peer group	Peer group	
	Local primarily	Local and distant	Local and distant
Roles	Mentee	Mentee	Mentee
	Peer mentor	Peer mentor	Peer mentor
	Mentor to trainees	Mentor to early-career faculty and trainees	Mentor to early- and mid-career faculty; and trainees

turn to each other for support and advice. Faculty also shift in their relationship with the mentorship process, starting first primarily as mentee in the early-career stage and then increasingly taking on the mentor role for other faculty in the mid-career- and advanced-career stages.

As mentioned previously, some faculty development content (eg, curricular innovations) is relevant to all faculty. There may be benefit in providing this content to all career stages through formal approaches. There may also be benefit in providing interventions for specific career stages, which may differ in the challenges of adapting to the new content.

There are significant limitations in the literature regarding faculty development at the different career stages. Most of the descriptions of programs and interventions focus on outcomes at the level of participant satisfaction and feasibility of implementation, with a few also involving more detailed analysis of qualitative data. How effective these programs are in terms of other outcomes is still relatively uncertain. The literature also becomes increasingly sparse toward the advanced-career stage, focusing primarily on needs assessment rather than descriptions and evaluations of specific interventions. Thus academic leaders are left with little guidance on what kinds of programs or interventions are going to be most helpful for faculty at the advanced-career stage.

In summary, a developmental approach to faculty development seems to increase the chances that programs and interventions will be more likely to meet the needs of faculty at different career stages. More work needs to be done to clearly establish the content and processes that will be most effective in faculty development initiatives at each career stage.

REFERENCES

1. Munley PH. Erikson's theory of psychosocial development and career development. J Vocat Behav 1977;10:261–9.
2. Levinson DJ, Darrow CN, Klein EB, et al. The seasons of a man's life. New York: Alfred A. Knopf; 1978.

3. Marcia JE, Waterman AS, Matteson DR, et al. Ego identity: a handbook for psychosocial research. New York: Springer-Verlag; 2012.

4. Bourgeois JA, Servis M. Clinical habits and the psychiatrist: an adult developmental model focusing on the academic psychiatrist. Acad Psychiatry 2006;30: 365–71.

5. Kanter SL. Faculty career progression. Acad Med 2011;86:919.

6. Silver I. Starting a faculty development program. In: Steinert Y, editor. Faculty development in the health professions: a focus on research and practice. New York: Springer; 2014. p. 331–49.

7. Leslie K. Faculty development for academic and career development. In: Steinert Y, editor. Faculty development in the health professions: a focus on research and practice. New York: Springer; 2014. p. 97–118.

8. Block SM, Sonnino RE, Bellini L. Defining "faculty" in academic medicine: responding to the challenges of a changing environment. Acad Med 2015;90: 279–82.

9. Jeanmonod R. Retaining talent at academic medical centers. Int J Acad Med 2016;2:46–51.

10. Cropsey KL, Masho SW, Shiang R, Committee on the Status of Women and Minorities, Virginia Commonwealth University School of Medicine, Medical College of Virginia Campus, et al. Why do faculty leave? Reasons for attrition of women and minority faculty from a medical school: four-year results. J Womens Health (Larchmt) 2008;17:1111–8.

11. Jackson VA, Palepu A, Szalacha L, et al. "Having the right chemistry": a qualitative study of mentoring in academic medicine. Acad Med 2003;78:328–34.

12. Bucklin BA, Valley M, Welch C, et al. Predictors of early faculty attrition at one academic medical center. BMC Med Educ 2014;14:27.

13. Steele M, Fisman S, Davidson B. Mentoring and role models in recruitment and retention: a study of junior medical faculty perceptions. Med Teach 2013;35(5): e1130–8.

14. Thorndyke LT, Gusic ME, George JH, et al. Empowering junior faculty: Penn State's faculty development and mentoring program. Acad Med 2006;81:668–73.

15. Pololi L, Knight S. Mentoring faculty in academic medicine. J Gen Intern Med 2005;20:866–70.

16. Palepu A, Friedman RH, Barnett RC, et al. Junior faculty members' mentoring relationships and their professional development in U.S. medical schools. Acad Med 1998;73:318–23.

17. Moss J, Teshima J, Leszcz M. Peer group mentoring of junior faculty. Acad Psychiatry 2008;32:230–5.

18. Lord JA, Mourtzanos E, McLaren K, et al. A peer mentoring group for junior clinician educators – four years' experience. Acad Med 2012;87:378–83.

19. Seritan AL, Bhangoo R, Garma S, et al. Society for women in academic psychiatry: a peer mentoring approach. Acad Psychiatry 2007;31:363–6.

20. Clark T, Corral J, Nyberg E, et al. Launchpad for onboarding new faculty into academic life. Curr Probl Diagn Radiol 2018;47:72–4.

21. Guillet R, Holloway RG, Gross RA, et al. Junior faculty core curriculum to enhance faculty development. J Clin Transl Sci 2017;1:77–82.

22. Pololi LH, Knight SM, Dennis K, et al. Helping medical school faculty realize their dreams: an innovative, collaborative mentoring program. Acad Med 2002;77: 377–84.

23. Ansmann L, Flickinger TE, Barello S, et al. Career development for early career academics: benefits of networking and the role of professional societies. Patient Educ Couns 2014;97:132–4.

24. Teruya SA, Bazargan-Hejazi S. Social media and mentoring in biomedical research faculty development. J Fac Dev 2014;28:13–22.

25. Blickle G, Witzki AH, Schneider PB. Mentoring support and power: a three year predictive field study on protégé networking and career success. J Vocat Behav 2009;74:181–9.

26. Forret ML, Dougherty TW. Networking behaviors and career outcomes: differences for men and women? J Organ Behav 2004;25:419–37.

27. Steinert Y, Naismith L, Mann K. Faculty development initiatives designed to promote leadership in medical education. A BEME systematic review: BEME Guide No. 19. Med Teach 2012;34:483–503.

28. Leslie K, Baker L, Egan-Lee E, et al. Advancing faculty development in medical education: a systematic review. Acad Med 2013;88:1038–45.

29. Helitzer DL, Newbill SL, Cardinali G, et al. Narratives of participants in national career development programs for women in academic medicine: identifying the opportunities for strategic investment. J Womens Health (Larchmt) 2016;25: 360–70.

30. Steinert Y, Mann K, Anderson B, et al. A systematic review of faculty development initiatives designed to enhance teaching effectiveness: a 10-year update: BEME Guide No. 40. Med Teach 2016;38:769–86.

31. Blitzstein S, Seritan A, Sockalingham S, et al. From industry to generativity: the first twelve years of the Association for Academic Psychiatry Master Educator Program. Acad Psychiatry 2016;40:576–83.

32. Tekian A, Harris I. Preparing health professions education leaders worldwide: a description of masters-level programs. Med Teach 2012;34:52–8.

33. Rayburn W, Grigsby K, Brubaker L. The strategic value of succession planning for department chairs. Acad Med 2016;91:465–8.

34. Spickard A, Gabbe SG, Christensen JF. Mid-career burnout in generalist and specialist physicians. JAMA 2002;288:1446–50.

35. Seritan AL. How to recognize and avoid burnout. In: Roberts LW, editor. Achievement and fulfillment in academic medicine: a comprehensive guide. New York: Springer; 2013. p. 447–54.

36. Hewlett SA, Luce CB. Off-ramps and on-ramps: keeping talented women on the road to success. Harv Bus Rev 2005;83:43–54.

37. Valantine HA, Grewal D, Ku MC, et al. The gender gap in academic medicine: comparing results from a multifaceted intervention for Stanford faculty to peer and national cohorts. Acad Med 2014;89:904–11.

38. Carnes M, Devine PG, Baier Manwell L, et al. The effect of an intervention to break the gender bias habit for faculty at one institution: a cluster randomized, controlled trial. Acad Med 2015;90:221–30.

39. Moss-Racusin CA, van der Toorn J, Dovidio JF, et al. Social science. Scientific diversity interventions. Science 2014;343:615–6.

40. Dannels SA, Yamagata H, McDade SA, et al. Evaluating a leadership program: a comparative, longitudinal study to assess the impact of the Executive Leadership in Academic Medicine (ELAM) Program for Women. Acad Med 2008;83:488–95.

41. McDade SA, Richman RC, Jackson GB, et al. Effects of participation in the Executive Leadership in Academic Medicine (ELAM) program on women faculty's perceived leadership capabilities. Acad Med 2004;79:302–9.

42. Bland CJ, Bergquist WH. The vitality of senior faculty members: snow on the roof-fire in the furnace. Washington, DC: George Washington University; 1997.
43. Daneman D, Kellner J. Navigating the stages of an academic career for paediatricians. Paediatr Child Health 2012;17(6):301–3.
44. Kram KE. Mentoring at work: developmental relationships in organizational life. Glenview (IL): Scott, Foresman, and Company; 1985.
45. Wakefield DS, Kienzle MG, Zollo SA, et al. Health care providers' perceptions of telemedicine services. Telemed J 1997;3(1):59–65.
46. Xu X, Schneider M, DeSorbo-Quinn AL, et al. Distance mentoring of health researchers: three case studies across the career-development trajectory. Health Psychol Open 2017;4(2). 2055102917734388.
47. Nivet MA. A diversity 3.0 update: are we moving the needle enough? Acad Med 2015;90(12):1591–3.
48. Mennin S, Kalishman S, Eklund MA, et al. Project-based faculty development by international health professions educators: practical strategies. Med Teach 2013; 35(2):e971–7.
49. Sorcinelli MD, Audstin AE, Eddy PL, et al. Creating the future of faculty development: learning from the past, understanding the present. San Francisco (CA): Jossey-Bass; 2006.
50. Onyura B, Bohnen J, Wasylenki D, et al. Reimagining the self at late-career transitions: how identity threat influences academic physicians' retirement considerations. Acad Med 2015;90(6):794–801.
51. Sonnino RE, Reznik V, Thorndyke LA, et al. Evolution of faculty affairs and faculty development offices in U.S. medical schools: a 10-year follow-up survey. Acad Med 2013;88(9):1368–75.

Professional Development for Clinical Faculty in Academia
Focus on Teaching, Research, and Leadership

Douglas Ziedonis, MD, MPH*, Mary S. Ahn, MD

KEYWORDS

- Professional development • Career development • Mentoring • Leadership
- Research • Teaching

KEY POINTS

- Professional development for clinical faculty in academic health centers is critical for improving their leadership, clinical practice, teaching, and scholarship skills.
- Protected time, training opportunities, access to mentors, and project resources can reduce commonly perceived barriers and challenges.
- Strategic alignment of faculty needs and institutional goals and priorities is vital and helps build teamwork and engagement.
- Aligning departmental and institutional professional development activities helps increase creativity, cross-departmental learning, and limited resources efficiencies.

INTRODUCTION

Professional development of clinical faculty is a key strategy in both supporting individual aspirations and the goals of academic health centers and departments. Creative, systematic, and supportive approaches help enhance individual faculty skills with the potential to enhance teamwork and institutional performance, engagement, and alignment. Clinical faculty are faced with increased clinical practice time demands and less time for academic interests and home life. Having protected time to attend the training activities that faculty want and see relevance in their work roles helps faculty members feel valued, heard, and supported. Successful models offer formal and informal programs with a range of mentoring and coaching options, including peer mentorship. Reducing burnout and disengagement can be supported through the

Disclosure Statement: M.S. Ahn: Principal and Owner, Life Sciences and Talent Development, PLLC. D. Ziedonis: None.
University of California San Diego, Biomedical Sciences Building, 9500 Gilman Drive #0602, La Jolla, CA 92093-0602, USA
* Corresponding author.
E-mail address: dziedonis@ucsd.edu

Psychiatr Clin N Am 42 (2019) 389–399
https://doi.org/10.1016/j.psc.2019.05.009
0193-953X/19/© 2019 Elsevier Inc. All rights reserved.

teambuilding aspects of these programs, addressing systemic factors as well as personal development to enhance resilience and leadership skills.

This article reviews professional development issues from the literature and summarizes a range of practical strategies for both individuals and institutions, including educational research studies of the impact of mentoring, leadership, education skill development, and peer coaching programs. As a case example, lessons learned from applying these strategies are described in one Psychiatry Department's Career Development and Research Office (CDRO). This article considers several questions:

1. What are common professional development priorities and how are they similar or different from the perspective of the individual, department, or institution?
2. What strategies can address the barriers and challenges to implementing professional development activities?
3. What national organizational resources can support local efforts to help clinical faculty with their professional development goals?

CLARIFYING PRIORITIES AND GOALS

Professional development priorities reflect the core values, aspirations, and needs of individuals, departments, and institutions. Commonly professional development will cover all 3 core mission areas (clinical, teaching, and scholarship) and also may include leadership and management skill development. Mission-based training must consider the institutional context and the faculty members' prior experience, skill level, role, and phase of career. Clinical faculty are commonly clinical employees of a clinical system and academic faculty of a university where the clinical and academic systems often have different and competing priorities and expectations for balancing teaching, scholarship, and service. Clinical faculty from different institutions often have varying academic promotion requirements, including tenure potential. This consideration will influence professional development needs and goals. Identifying and supporting professional development needs starts in the recruitment and hiring process and continues with onboarding, orientation, and networking into the community and culture of the institution. Individual professional development plans and connections with supervisors and mentors can help them identify areas of interest, need, and priority.

PROFESSIONAL DEVELOPMENT AND A CAREER DEVELOPMENT PLAN

Clinical faculty can benefit from mentorship and career coaching that helps them create an evolving career development plan. This is a personal process that requires self-reflection, competing life priorities, and realistic assessment of current strengths and areas for growth. In the context of developing a career development plan, clinical faculty have an opportunity to ask themselves major questions such as:

- Where would they like to make a difference?
- What is important for them at this time of their life and career?
- What brings them joy and fulfillment in their life?

The answer to these questions may align well with their current job and their employer's interests, or not. This is a time for individuals to consider how to best align their goals and priorities with their employer's and work team, including what their strengths are and where their opportunities are for growth. Asking for feedback from others can be done by the individual, or perhaps with the help of a coach, on how they are doing and where the opportunities exist for making a better impact. Creating a career development plan includes setting short-term and long-term goals and functionally matching each goal with the necessary professional development activity. The departmental annual performance evaluation is an opportunity for getting and giving feedback, including mentoring and career development needs.

PROFESSIONAL DEVELOPMENT FOR ENHANCING TEACHING SKILLS

Teaching medical students, residents, and other allied health students often occurs in a wide variety of settings and can provide an opportunity for interprofessional education using a range of teaching methods and pedagogy approaches. The Association of American Medical Colleges (AAMC), Accreditation Council for Graduate Medical Education, American Medical Association, and other national medical education organizations provide competencies and professional development resources, training, and networking opportunities.

The AAMC's MedEdPortal (https://www.mededportal.org/) is a useful resource for creative and innovative ways to provide medical education. This site also provides an opportunity to encourage clinical faculty to share their own ideas and activities for medical education with many others, which is a way to expand their scholarship and impact on the field.

The Best Evidence Medical Education (BEME) Collaboration is an international organization that has conducted systematic literature reviews to create best-practice summaries to inform faculty development focused on improving teaching skills in medical education (https://www.bemecollaboration.org). In the past almost 20 years, there have been 42 Guides published in *Medical Teacher* in an effort to increase the evidence-based nature of professional development programs for medical education practice.[1] The Kirkpatrick model is one example of a commonly used methodology in evaluating educational programs along 4 levels of increasing impact, namely:

1. Reaction to the training such as the degree of satisfaction and attendance
2. Learning in the session assessing attitudes, skills, and knowledge change
3. Behavior in the work context using the new skills or knowledge learned in the program
4. Results of the impact of using the new skills and knowledge on patients, organizations, teams, and so forth

A BEME summary analysis of the faculty developer's competences as facilitators in professional development programs identified negotiating, constructing, and attuning as critical in understanding the context of the training.[2] A BEME systematic review of faculty development to improve medical education teaching used the Kirkpatrick 4 outcome levels for 53 studies, including 6 being randomized controlled trials,[3] and confirmed that the key effective components of the training were using the principles of adult learning,[4] experiential learning,[5] peer support, well-designed training programs, and multiple educational methods.[3] In addition, professional development to promote leadership in medical education was systematically reviewed by BEME,[6] using 48 articles and 35 interventions, whereby it was found that leadership training programs were often short (less than 3.5 days); however, longer training may have better outcomes and included a wider range of leadership topics (eg, conflict management, finance, team building, people management), a system-level focus (change management), and career planning. Some key aspects of effective programs were including multiple teaching methods, experiential learning, time for reflections, both individual and group projects based in the faculty's real-world roles, and components of peer support, mentorship, and institutional support.[6]

There is still a need to develop and evaluate which methods would be most effective in different settings, different specialties, with simulation teaching and other educational technology, and with what outcomes.[7] Peer group mentoring may provide a cost-effective and powerfully supportive model to include in mentoring programs in addition to the more traditional dyad mentor-mentee model.[8] Peer mentoring has been used effectively in programs supporting women, minority faculty, and junior faculty, including better addressing challenges and barriers of competing responsibilities, accountability, selection of senior advisors, and finding a common interest.[9] Developing mentoring competencies is an important skill that is often untaught. Even a single half-day of evidence-based training on how to be a mentor can make an impact.[10] The Mentoring Competency Assessment tool with 26 items can be used to assess mentors' competencies, including addressing different gender, cultural, and generational background perspectives.[11]

New ways of engaging faculty are being implemented with social media, including the use of Twitter. This is a method used to address barriers of funding and limited resources. Using this platform for professional development has found that networks can be expanded and can help with communication skills, increase knowledge in peer-supported and self-directed manner, and provide new opportunities for professional growth.[12]

PROFESSIONAL DEVELOPMENT FOR LEADERSHIP AND MANAGEMENT

The American College of Healthcare Executives (ACHE) Competencies Assessment Tool is useful for self-assessments and for developing a leadership career development plan. The tool is available free at http://www.ache.org/pdf/nonsecure/careers/competencies_booklet.pdf. The online tool was developed from surveys by the Healthcare Leadership Alliance and assesses 5 competency areas: Leadership, Communication & Relationship Management, Professionalism, Knowledge of the Healthcare Environment, and Business Skills and Knowledge. Self-assessment by faculty of their own ability to independently identify their own needs does not yet have a strong research database to support this; however, departmental and/or institutional engagement in the process might help, especially with support, multiple other inputs of feedback, follow-up, and agreeing to the value of the standards and competencies.[13]

Professional development programs to improve leadership skills are critical and can help align individual, departmental, and institutional needs and goals. Leadership skills are different from management skills and include creating a shared vision, inspiring others, assessing climate and culture, communication, change management, creating an environment of mutual trust, and supporting others in their leadership work. The balance of management and leadership skills will vary by role, including whether front-line, middle management, or higher-level leadership. Leadership is needed to help support clinical faculty and others' wellness through health promotion.[14] Mindfulness-oriented professional development training can be helpful for increasing communication skills, self-compassion leading to compassion for others, being more self-aware, and increasing focus in the present moment.[15–17] Communication skill development will help in all mission areas through improving listening skills, self-awareness, written/oral communication messaging by tailoring to the audience, managing relationships, facilitating discussions in groups, respectful communication, inclusive excellence, allyship, and bystander intervention.[18–26]

The Stanford Leadership Development program learning model has been described and evaluated as showing how leadership training for clinician leaders can be effective.[27] The Stanford program occurred over a 9-month time period and is an excellent example of covering a wide range of leadership topics, and included multiple adult learning methods, including an experiential leadership project. The Kirkpatrick assessment levels were used to evaluate the program and found high participation levels, satisfaction, and improvement in attitudes, skills, and knowledge on leadership competencies, engaged in a leadership project using these skills, and successfully completed their team-based project https://www.kirkpatrickpartners.com. The program used the Activation-Demonstration-Application-Integration education training framework[28] of effective education.[27]

Professional development leadership courses are available by most national professional organizations and also present a great opportunity for local institutions to offer while combining local change management and strategic planning. Most of the national professional organizations have an Annual Meeting, Secondary Meetings of key professional development groups, conferences, Web site/online resources, and written materials. For example, The AAMC offers 18 different professional development groups to help with networking, peer to peer support, leadership, interprofessionalism, and ways to stay current in specific areas (https://www.aamc.org/). Examples relevant to clinical faculty include Chief Medical Officers Group, Group on Faculty Practice, Group on Educational Affairs, Group on Student Affairs, and Group on Diversity and Inclusion. The AAMC offers numerous leadership development and certification programs for all phases of individuals' careers and roles, including leading information technology in academic medicine, health care diversity and inclusion, conflict management, early and mid-career women faculty leadership development, leadership and management foundations for Academic Medicine and Sciences, GME leadership, CMOs, New Deans, Associate Deans, and Chairs training.

PROFESSIONAL DEVELOPMENT FOR RESEARCH AND ACADEMIC SCHOLARSHIP

Mentoring is an important method for supporting careers in research and medical education.[7,29,30] Academic departments commonly have identified mentors, and there is a growing body of literature on effective mentoring programs and techniques. For example, the University of Wisconsin's ICTR is leading a National Research Mentoring Network with numerous training programs and also a core team that is developing, evaluating, and disseminating evidence-based curriculum (https://ictr.wisc.edu/mentoring/).[31–35] Effective mentoring has been critical for most researchers in academic medicine, but also important for clinical, teaching, and leadership professional development. This research group has developed the Center for the Improvement of Mentored Experiences in Research (CIMER), which provides useful resources to train both mentors and mentees at all career stages for research career development, including building a network of individuals and institutions. Resources are available at https://cimerproject.org/#/curricula/training-materials. Mentoring programs commonly provide advice on selecting a mentor (often multiple mentors, peer-mentors, or mentors within and outside of an organization), establishing a written agreement on the mentor-mentee relationship, roles and expectations for both, and ways to evaluate the effectiveness of the relationship, including the ability of the mentee to achieve his or her goals.[36,37] The CIMER group has developed the Mentoring Competency Assessment, which includes 26 mentoring skills items, including maintaining effective communication, aligning expectations, assessing understanding, addressing diversity, fostering independence, and promoting professional development.[11]

CASE EXAMPLE OF THE UMass DEPARTMENT OF PSYCHIATRY

Individual faculty members have unique needs and aspirations that will benefit from institutional support and aligning with the priorities of the institution. Each academic health center and department has its own unique history, culture, priorities, resources, and leadership challenges and opportunities; however, Chairs and other system leaders must act and decide how to support professional development for their clinical faculty. This article concludes with an example of how one psychiatry department in transition with a new Chair responded to these needs within the context of its system.

The department was large at baseline (225 faculty) and had strengths in most mission areas; however, there were institutional expectations to increase the clinical research activity and productivity while strengthening the educational and clinical missions. From a faculty needs assessment survey, numerous focus groups, and department inclusive strategic planning process, the leaders identified a strong interest and need to "Develop the Workforce of the Future":

1. Offer career and research mentors and programs
2. Reduce intradepartmental silos
3. Build infrastructure support, including protected time for professional development and scholarship and resources for starting research projects
4. Assist with the academic promotion process

In response, departmental leaders developed a CDRO, which offered a variety of resources to meet the diverse needs of the large faculty body and worked closely with the institution's Office of Faculty Affairs, which had varying levels of annual funding support. On inception, the CDRO aimed to support a culture of mentoring, including individual, peer, and team mentoring.

Both formal and informal needs assessments obtained from individual faculty members were conducted through the annual performance evaluation (there were specific sections dedicated to elicit information about needs for mentoring and career development, in alignment with the department's strategic plan). In addition, the faculty was engaged as a whole through the annual departmental meetings of the department's strategic plan, which included "Developing a Workforce of the Future" as 1 of the 5 major strategic priority areas. Lastly, the CDRO's annual faculty needs assessment survey guided the plans for the catalog of professional development programs. In turn, annually a systematic review of both departmental and institutional programs and supports were reviewed and cataloged for use by both faculty and their supervisors.

The primary mission of the CDRO was to help each individual faculty member achieve excellence through access and support of learning communities, scholarship, professional development, and mentoring across the full range of faculty interests and stages in the career life cycle, including support for academic skills, promotion, and career advancement. The CDRO services included one-on- one coaching meetings with CDRO staff for promotion guidance, budget planning, recruitment issues, funding identification, and overall research or career development support. All new faculty offer letters provided information about the CDRO and connected them to a mentor and the CDRO as part of the onboarding process.

Mentoring was a key professional development component targeting leadership, teaching, and research. The CDRO developed mentoring training programs (including a New Faculty onboarding program), peer coaching support (including a Women's Faculty Committee), and a leadership development program, entitled the Leadership College.[38] Clinical faculty also sought out mentoring on academic promotion, including resumé enhancement, writing the necessary support documents, and putting together their packet. The CDRO developed rank-specific seminars on achieving promotion, as well as providing individual consultation. In addition, support for clinical faculty included outreach to their workplace, engaging all team members and their respective leaders to address barriers and challenges and to receive both ideas and feedback on how the department could be a resource to their direct workplace.

Academic Interest Groups were also developed to help increase faculty with a common interest (including clinical and research-oriented faculty, basic and clinical faculty, students, and staff) which provided an opportunity for networking and to support professional development, mentoring, and team building. The CDRO supported the Academic Interest Groups as a way to increase collaborations and reduce silos across the department. The CDRO provided support for coordinating monthly meetings, providing updates on relevant funding opportunities, and connecting with institutional resources. These groups would provide updates to the CDRO on their activities, and the groups and their leaders were recognized and honored at an annual reception with award recognition activities.

To support professional development in research, the CDRO provided support with IRB submissions, recruitment of research subjects, and handling the administrative side of running a research project or program. In addition, several writing groups were formed, including a very successful NIH "K Award writing group" developed for clinical faculty committed to an independent investigator research career. The CDRO also hosted an annual Psychiatry Research Day, a day-long event of presentations, peer-reviewed poster sessions, awards, and a high-profile keynote speaker (eg, Directors of NIDA, NIMH, NCCAM, SAMHSA, Research on Women's Health, PCORI). Clinical faculty might have a poster that described their clinical setting and population receiving care, which led to new collaborations with established research-oriented faculty.

In its most recent evolution, the CDRO has used internal coaching to support faculty in a confidential setting. Departmental faculty either self-refer or are referred by their supervisors, but the service is entirely voluntary and confidential. Areas covered include career coaching, leadership coaching, or performance coaching, which target specific skills to be improved. All of the coaching was done by 2 internal faculty coaches who were credentialed by the International Coach Federation and/or the Worldwide Association of Business Coaches, who were also certified in several coaching instruments to facilitate self- and other-awareness, such as the DiSC (https://www.discprofile.com) for work productivity, teamwork, and communication skills and the Eq-I 2.0 (https://www.mhs.com/MHS-Talent) for emotional intelligence. Also, 360° assessments (https://www.echospan.com/360-degree-feedback-landing. asp) (both through formal and informal assessments) were used to facilitate insight and establish coaching goals. Because the internal coaches were departmental faculty, they had the unique knowledge and skill set to understand the faculty member's workplace environment and unique history and culture of the department as well as the broader system.

No doubt the CDRO will continue to evolve in response to the changing landscape of the department and the needs of their faculty. After the first 10 years of CDRO support, the department grew in size from about 225 faculty to over 380, and dramatically increased activities and impact in research, education, wellness, leadership, and clinical services.

Table 1
Best practices or interventions for professional development

Approach	Brief Description	Comments
Peer mentoring training and developing a learning community	Initially trains the peer group on mentoring and coaching skills and includes a planned curriculum; institutionally supported with protected time	9 mo to 1 y within 1 department or across the institution
Mentorship training and matching Programs	Matches mentee faculty to mentor faculty; includes support/structure to enhance mentor and mentee effectiveness. Varies by mission area focus and established goals	Mentoring becomes part of culture and processes
Institutional support for professional development	Provides protected time and project funds while engaging senior leadership, recognition for those involved, linkages to future leadership roles	Varies by institution and department in amount of time and resources
Multiple instructional methods in delivering these programs	Uses adult learning methods, including small group discussions, role plays, simulations, interactive learning experiences, reflective practice.	Vary by number of methods used and theoretic models used
Individual and team or group projects	Applies new knowledge and skills addressing real-world problems in the participants' direct workplace setting	Time, project funds, and recognition can accelerate positive outcomes
Career promotion workshops	Guides faculty to advance their career with multiple pathways/mechanisms to create scholarship in academic medicine	Career Development Plan training
Teaching skills workshops	Enhances communication, instructional, technology, and curriculum development skills	Feedback on observed teaching; simulation
Leadership courses and programs	Enhances self-awareness, uses assessment tools (eg, 360, DiSC), teaches management and leadership skills development	Aligns with participant's current or future projects and roles
AAMC MedEdPortal	Offers training to access and contribute to one's own scholarship	www.mededportal.org/
Leadership College, UMass Department of Psychiatry	Uses facilitated peer coaching; assesses emotional intelligence (EQI2), communication, and negotiation skills and systems awareness; uses ACHE leadership competencies assessment tool	Part of the Career Development and Research Office (CDRO)[38]
Mindful physician leadership program	www.umassmed.edu/psychiatry/education/mindfulphysician leadershipprogram/	Foundational, Advanced, and Train-the-trainer levels[16,17]

(continued on next page)

Table 1 *(continued)*		
Approach	**Brief Description**	**Comments**
Stanford leadership development program	https://med.stanford.edu/faculty diversity/faculty-development/ leadership-programs/stanford- leadership-develop-program.html	
University of Wisconsin's CIMER training program	https://cimerproject.org/#/curricula/ training-materials	Training materials and National Research Mentoring Network
K Award writing group	Research Career Award writing group for NIH, VA, and other training grants	

Data from Steinert Y, Mann K, Centeno A, et al. A systematic review of faculty development initiatives designed to improve teaching effectiveness in medical education: BEME Guide No. 8. Med Teach 2006;28(6):497–526; and Steinert Y, Naismith L, Mann K. Faculty development initiatives designed to promote leadership in medical education. A BEME systematic review: BEME Guide No. 19. Med Teach 2012;34(6):483–503.

SUMMARY

The risk for burnout, disengagement, and feeling overwhelmed has increased with more time demands from clinical practice and less time to teach, lead, or innovate. Academic institutions and departments have a unique opportunity to engage its faculty by sponsoring and creating innovative professional development programs to enhance leadership, research, teaching, and clinical skills. The added benefit of these "homegrown" programs is that the clinical faculty members feel more valued, engaged, and supported and will want to better align their priorities with the strategic priorities of the institution. There are excellent national resources to support and complement local professional development efforts. There are best practices and some standard approaches to learn from nationally; however, each department needs to balance any standard with customized approaches (**Table 1**).

Clinical faculty need creative, systematic, and supportive approaches to help their career and professional development. Listening to their needs and concerns is vital in developing these programs. There are many national, institutional, and departmental best practices that can be sources of new ways to expand offerings locally or to provide opportunities to go and attend. Academic institutions and their departments have a unique opportunity to engage its faculty by sponsoring and creating innovative professional development programs to enhance leadership, research, teaching, and clinical skills. The added benefit of these "homegrown" programs is that clinical faculty members will feel more valued as individuals, engaged, and supported to want to align their priorities with the strategic priorities of the institution. Protected time to take part in these programs and activities respects the reality of clinical faculty's busy clinical practice schedules that have limited time for teaching and scholarly activities. There are excellent national resources to support and complement these professional development efforts.

REFERENCES

1. Maggio LA, Thomas A, Chen HC, et al. Examining the readiness of best evidence in medical education guides for integration into educational practice: a meta-synthesis. Perspect Med Educ 2018;7(5):292–301.

2. Baker L, Leslie K, Panisko D, et al. Exploring faculty developers' experiences to inform our understanding of competence in faculty development. Acad Med 2018;93(2):265–73.

3. Steinert Y, Mann K, Centeno A, et al. A systematic review of faculty development initiatives designed to improve teaching effectiveness in medical education: Best Evidence Medical and Health Professional Education (BEME) Guide No. 8. Med Teach 2006;28(6):497–526.

4. Knowles MS, Holton EF III, Swanson RA. The adult learner. New York: Routledge; 2012.

5. Kolb AY, Kolb DA. Learning styles and learning spaces: enhancing experiential learning in higher education. Acad Manag Learn Educ 2005;4(2):193–212.

6. Steinert Y, Naismith L, Mann K. Faculty development initiatives designed to promote leadership in medical education. A Best Evidence Medical and Health Professional Education (BEME) systematic review: BEME Guide No. 19. Med Teach 2012;34(6):483–503.

7. Farrell SE, Digioia NM, Broderick KB, et al. Mentoring for clinician-educators. Acad Emerg Med 2004;11(12):1346–50.

8. Moss J, Teshima J, Leszcz M. Peer group mentoring of junior faculty. Acad Psychiatry 2008;32(3):230–5.

9. Bussey-Jones J, Bernstein L, Higgins S, et al. Repaving the road to academic success: the IMeRGE approach to peer mentoring. Acad Med 2006;81(7):674–9.

10. Lau C, Ford J, Van Lieshout RJ, et al. Developing mentoring competency: does a one session training workshop have impact? Acad Psychiatry 2016;40(3):429–33.

11. Fleming M, House MS, Shewakramani MV, et al. The mentoring competency assessment: validation of a new instrument to evaluate skills of research mentors. Acad Med 2013;88(7):1002.

12. Hart M, Stetten NE, Islam S, et al. Twitter and public health (part 1): how individual public health professionals use twitter for professional development. JMIR Public Health Surveill 2017;3(3):e60.

13. Colthart I, Bagnall G, Evans A, et al. The effectiveness of self-assessment on the identification of learner needs, learner activity, and impact on clinical practice: BEME Guide No. 10. Med Teach 2008;30(2):124–45.

14. Hoert J, Herd AM, Hambrick M. The role of leadership support for health promotion in employee wellness program participation, perceived job stress, and health behaviors. Am J Health Promot 2018;32(4):1054–61.

15. Marturano J. Finding the space to lead: a practical guide to mindful leadership. New York: Bloomsbury Publishing; 2014.

16. Ziedonis D, Fulwiler C, Tonelli M. Integrating mindfulness into your daily routine. Vital Signs 2014;19(2):6.

17. Tonelli M, Fulwiler C, de Torrijos F, et al. Mindfulness in psychiatry program and emerging initiatives at the University of Massachusetts & UMass Memorial Health Care. Worcester Med 2016;80(2):14–5.

18. Lieff SJ, Yammarino FJ. How to lead the way through complexity, constraint, and uncertainty in academic health science centers. Acad Med 2017;92(5):614–21.

19. West M, Armit K, Loewenthal L, et al. Leadership and leadership development in healthcare: the evidence base. London: The Kings Fund; 2015.

20. Stefl ME. Common competencies for all healthcare managers: the Healthcare Leadership Alliance model. J Healthc Manag 2008;53(6):360–73.

21. Stefl ME. Expert leaders for healthcare administration. Healthc Pap 2003;4(1):59–90.

22. Rice JA. Investing in the three Rs. Developing physician leadership to help hospitals achieve success. Healthc Exec 2007;22(6):56–60.
23. Rice JA. Governing a new generation of philanthropy: key leadership tools for success. AHP J 2008;(8-9):11–2.
24. Rice JA. Career and competency mapping. Leaders embrace life-long learning for success. Healthc Exec 2006;21(6):52–5.
25. Rice JA. Investing in physician leadership academies. Aligned interests among physicians and hospitals demand a new cadre of physician leaders. Healthc Exec 2009;24(2):64–5, 67.
26. Daly J, Jackson D, Mannix J, et al. The importance of clinical leadership in the hospital setting. J Healthc Leadersh 2014;6:75–83.
27. Hopkins J, Fassiotto M, Ku MC, et al. Designing a physician leadership development program based on effective models of physician education. Health Care Manage Rev 2018;43(4):293–302.
28. Merrill MD. First principles of instruction. Educ Technol Res Dev 2002;50(3): 43–59.
29. Sambunjak D, Straus SE, Marusic A. Mentoring in academic medicine: a systematic review. J Am Med Assoc 2006;296(9):1103–15.
30. Hafsteinsdóttir TB, van der Zwaag AM, Schuurmans MJ. Leadership mentoring in nursing research, career development and scholarly productivity: a systematic review. Int J Nurs Stud 2017;75:21–34.
31. Pfund C, Spencer KC, Asquith P, et al. Building national capacity for research mentor training: an evidence-based approach to training the trainers. CBE Life Sci Educ 2015;14(2):1–12.
32. Pfund C, House S, Spencer K, et al. A research mentor training curriculum for clinical and translational researchers. Clin Transl Sci 2013;6(1):26–33.
33. Pfund C, House SC, Asquith P, et al. Training mentors of clinical and translational research scholars: a randomized controlled trial. Acad Med 2014;89(5):774.
34. Feldman MD, Huang L, Guglielmo BJ, et al. Training the next generation of research mentors: the University of California, San Francisco, clinical & translational science institute mentor development program. Clin Transl Sci 2009;2(3): 216–21.
35. Byars-Winston AM, Branchaw J, Pfund C, et al. Culturally diverse undergraduate researchers' academic outcomes and perceptions of their research mentoring relationships. Int J Sci Educ 2015;37(15):2533–54.
36. Meagher E, Taylor L, Probsfield J, et al. Evaluating research mentors working in the area of clinical translational science: a review of the literature. Clin Transl Sci 2011;4(5):353–8.
37. Pfund C, Maidl Pribbenow C, Branchaw J, et al. Professional skills. The merits of training mentors. Science 2006;311(5760):473–4.
38. Ahn M. Leadership Agility Training: building emotional intelligence through peer coaching. Podium presentation presented at the Association of American Medical Colleges Group on Faculty Affairs Professional Development Conference, July 28, 2017, Vancouver, BC, Canada.

Coaching Health Care Leaders and Teams in Psychiatry

Mary S. Ahn, MD[a],*, Douglas Ziedonis, MD, MPH[b]

KEYWORDS

- Coaching • Mentoring • Leadership • Career development • Psychiatry

KEY POINTS

- The mentoring and coaching needs of leaders at all levels in behavioral health and psychiatry departments, services, and organizations have grown as the identity and roles of leaders in the profession have broadened and become more complex.
- There are several types of coaching used in health care, and they have distinctions from traditional mentoring and therapy, including clinical, transformational, wellness, business, and leadership coaching.
- Coaching is highly beneficial not only to the individuals in their leadership roles, but also in improving patient care, provider engagement, and team building.
- Coaching increases self-awareness, emotional intelligence, communication skills, and work-life balance through the relationship of the coach and the client, and with the help of coaching tools that include self and peer assessments.

INTRODUCTION

In recent years, increasing administrative and clinical demands have been placed on leaders in behavioral health and psychiatry departments, services, and organizations and their frontline clinicians to expand patient-centered team-based care to improve patient adherence to treatment, patient satisfaction, and the provision of cost-effective care in the era of the electronic medical record and shorter patient encounters. Some of these organizations will be in complex larger systems in which academic and community engagement missions are vital. Creating influence is an essential leadership skill in the context of limited authority over direct decisions in a

Disclosure Statement: M.S. Ahn: Principal and Owner, Life Sciences and Talent Development, PLLC. D. Ziedonis: None.
[a] Department of Psychiatry, University of Massachusetts Medical School, 55 Lake Avenue North, Worcester, MA 01655-0002, USA; [b] University of California San Diego, UC San Diego Health, Biomedical Sciences Building, 9500 Gilman Drive #0602, La Jolla, CA 92093-0602, USA
* Corresponding author.
E-mail address: Mary.Ahn@umassmed.edu

climate of increasing regulations and compliance issues. In addition, clinician leaders who are practicing within this changing landscape are increasingly seeking out opportunities to become administrative leaders in health care, academic, and government agencies. For physicians, leadership skills are often not taught in medical school or in residency or fellowship training, as they are not considered core competencies in graduate medical education in psychiatry.

Coaching is now part of the professional development of leaders in many other businesses and industry sectors. Health care organizations have more slowly embraced coaching unless there is a perceived problem leader who is in trouble and needs to increase self-awareness of their impact on others and improve interpersonal and leadership skills. Coaching is now becoming more common in health care and academic settings, and there is a changing culture of hiring external coaches or developing internal coaching programs as part of leadership development and addressing concerns. Understandably, clinical and academic leaders are often selected for their expertise in clinical, research, or education, but not leadership skills. They are often quickly promoted to leadership positions with limited onboarding or succession planning by the previous leaders. Furthermore, some individuals are recognized as potential leaders for their managerial or organizational skills and promoted without attention to their need for executive leadership skills (such as strategic planning, communication, negotiation, leading teams). In fact, 79% of health care organizations have been reported to not routinely include succession planning in their strategic plan.[1]

Coaches have knowledge of general leadership and management competencies; however, there are also unique needs and skills for leaders in health care settings that are useful. The need for leadership competencies for physicians has resulted in the American College of Healthcare Executives (ACHE) to publish a self-assessment tool for leaders to assess and integrate into their own individualized educational plans. The following 5 core leadership and management areas are identified in the ACHE tool:

a. Communication and relationship management
b. Leadership (eg, creating a vision, managing change, organizational climate/culture, growing human resources talent)
c. Professionalism
d. Knowledge of the health care environment
e. Business skills and knowledge[2]

To date, there is no current literature about coaching specific to psychiatrists or other leaders in behavioral health settings; the field of coaching in health care is only beginning to emerge. The initial data are promising in support of coaching in health care as a way to increase resiliency and prevent burnout in both health system leaders and frontline clinicians.[3] This article reviews key coaching concepts from the general coaching literature and describes how they can be adapted to coaching in behavioral health and psychiatry organizations, as well as presents how the authors have integrated coaching into their own personal work with others and into a large department of psychiatry. In addition, how coaching techniques can be integrated to enhance traditional mentoring programs in psychiatry are also described.

WHAT IS COACHING?

In the broadest definition, coaching is a form of accelerated, individualized learning that is a time-limited, client-centered intervention.[4] Learning goals are mutually agreed on by both the client and coach, with expected outcomes set to ensure accountability.

The practice of coaching and how it is implemented can be as diverse as the clients, depending on the goals and the type of coach that is engaged.

Unfortunately, to date, there is no single standard training or credentialing program required to become a coach. The most widely used global credentialing organization for coaching is the International Coach Federation (ICF), which provides independent certification for coaches. ICF accredits not only individual coaches for their knowledge, skills, training, and experience but also evaluates and accredits training programs that adhere to their strict core competencies and ethical standards. Increasingly, health care organizations are hiring specifically ICF-accredited coaches due to the high standards and evaluation that is required to become credentialed.[5] The ICF has identified 11 core coaching competencies: Meeting Ethical Guidelines and Professional Standards, Establishing the Coaching Agreement, Establishing Trust and Intimacy with the Client, Coaching Presence, Active Listening, Powerful Questioning, Direct Communication, Creating Awareness, Designing Actions, Planning and Goal Setting, and Managing Progress and Accountability. These competencies are divided into 4 categories (Setting the Foundation, Co-Creating the Relationship, Communicating Effectively, and Facilitating Learning and Results). There are 3 different levels of ICF certification (Associate, Professional, and Master Certified Coach) with primarily increasing levels of training hours and hours of paid coaching experience. More information is available at the ICF Web site: https://coachfederation.org/icf-credential.

Another example of an organization trying to improve standards and professionalism in the coaching field is the World Association of Business Coaches (WABC), which focuses primarily on business coaching. WABC has 3 core competency areas (Self-Management-Knowing Oneself and Self-Mastery, Core Coaching Skill-Base, and Business and Leadership Coaching Capabilities) and the specific coaching competencies in these 3 areas are described on their Web site: http://www.wabccoaches.com/includes/popups/competencies.html. Similar to ICF, WABC credentials individuals at increasing levels of coaching skill (Registered Corporate Coach, WABC Certified Business Coach, WABC Certified Master Business Coach, and Chartered Business Coach). In addition to ICF and WABC, other organizations have created competencies that have some overlap, but also some key differences. In addition, many experienced and reputable coaches have been engaged by many organizations as coaches for decades before the certification programs were developed; however, more of these coaches have decided to pursue certification in recent years. Although there is no current consensus on which pathway or credentialing approach is the ideal one, the Institute of Coaching (McLean Hospital, Harvard Medical School Affiliate), a nonprofit organization that leads the health care field in coaching research grants and its annual coaching meeting, recommends gaining credentialization and refers directly to the ICF for resources.

COACHING VERSUS MENTORING VERSUS THERAPY

Mentors have demonstrated success and can serve not only as educators but also as role models. There is also a growing evidence-based literature on the competencies of mentors and for mentees.[6,7] These experienced professionals are chosen as mentors for their expertise in a field, an organization, or a particular area of skill or knowledge for the mentee. For example, they may be experts in program development, research, teaching, schizophrenia, depression, or population health. There are endless possibilities of expertise. Mentors also must spend time cultivating their mentor relationship with mentees, including how they will interact, helping the mentee develop goals, teaching specific skills, and helping with career progression advice. Mentors often share their own personal experience in the targeted area, including technical skills, feedback and insights, and other expertise in addition to providing invaluable sponsorship and networking opportunities. Internal mentors also provide advice on workplace culture and politics, as well as organizational issues. Although the best mentors will provide some coaching, they are often too busy to thoroughly assume both roles. For those who have multiple roles with a particular individual, they will likely need to share what role they are in for different meetings (eg, supervisor, mentor, coach).

Coaches normally do not offer advice, opinions, or solutions or share their own experiences, in contrast to mentors. The focus is on the client. Coaches use active listening and powerful questions that create a catalyst for change and growth in self-awareness, other-awareness, and ultimately a change in behaviors. Coaching is best used for identifying both strengths to leverage as well as increasing insight into developmental areas for influence, such as communication, interpersonal skills, or resiliency training, while also being an accountability partner. Often, coaches are more readily available to clients (often via on-demand e-mail, text, video calling, or phone calls).

A mentee will benefit both personally and professionally from using BOTH coaches and mentors over the course of their professional career as they play different roles. A coach can reinforce skills learned through professional development activities offered by an organization by individualizing their needs and organize a career development plan by putting knowledge acquired into actionable goals and skills.[8]

The practice of coaching has considerable overlap with psychotherapy, but the two should be carefully held distinct. Although coaching incorporates positive psychology and some of the tenets of cognitive behavioral therapy, it should be very clear if one is working with a patient or client. As a physician who practices coaching, it is especially prudent to define the role and refer to a separate medical provider if psychiatric or other medical needs arise.

TYPES OF COACHING

Please refer to **Table 1**, which summarizes the types of coaching.

Clinical coaching in medicine has been described to develop faculty,[9,10] as well as medical students and residents.[11,12] Similar to a batting coach in baseball, clinical coaching consists of longitudinal supervision of a learner and is skills-based, incorporating both observation and offering feedback and practices to improve a technique. Quality improvement training incorporates these types of coaches. A recent multisite, multidisciplinary study of residency programs used the R2C2 model,[13] which consists of 4 phases:

- *Relationship* Building
- Exploring *Reactions*
- Exploring *Content*
- *Coaching*

The coaches were recruited from the existing pool of supervisors already conducting assessment and feedback sessions with the trainees. The R2C2 model seemed to engage residents to reflect seriously on their feedback and areas for improvement. This generally fostered mutually agreed on goals and motivation for change for skills improvement compared with providing feedback alone. One of the drawbacks of clinical coaching is the supervisory nature of the coach, which may limit the client's ability to be fully vulnerable and honest with the coach. Of note, clinical coaches are not recognized as coaching, as defined by ICF and WABC.

Table 1
Types of coaching

Type of Coaching	Description	Coach Attributes	Author Comments
Clinical coaching	Skills-based supervision to improve a medical technique	• Recruited based on their content experience in a particular skill • Often provide assessment for evaluation back to the training program	• Specific to heath care and medical education • Not recognized by coaching industry • Coaches providing their feedback not only to the individual but also to a training program can be problematic to the coach-client relationship
Performance coaching	Transformational coaching style focused on improving a specific developmental area for a client	• An open and trusting relationship between the client and coach is key • The coach must establish the communication strategy (ideally in writing) among the coach, client, and the sponsoring organization, when applicable	• Often a sponsoring organization will request some general feedback • Coaches are most successful when expectations of the sponsoring organization are clearly outlined • An initial consultation may be helpful to establish the "coachability" of the client and the client's motivation to improve
Career coaching	Transformational coaching style focused on creating insight and motivation for professional development	• Uses positive psychology techniques • Avoids giving direct advice • Connects (or reconnects) clients with their passion, strengths, and values	• Important for coaches to understand the career life cycle common in health care (ie, early, mid, and late career issues) • Although the focus is primarily professional, personal issues as they intersect with work are addressed as well

(continued on next page)

Table 1
(continued)

Type of Coaching	Description	Coach Attributes	Author Comments
Leadership coaching	Transformational coaching style to develop leadership attributes necessary to take on a leadership role	• A self-assessment or 360 assessment of leadership competencies (ie, American College of Healthcare Executives) can establish the coaching needs of the individual leader	• Although coaches need not have the leadership experience that parallel the client's experience, some direct health care leadership experience in health care is preferred and sought-after
Business coaching	Transformational coaching style to align individual self-awareness with business acumen (often in their current place of employment)	• Can be individual or team-based	• Most coaches are sought-after for their direct experience in entrepreneurial or business ventures
Health and wellness coaching	Transformational coaching style to assist health care providers on their own self-care and/or how to educate their patients	• Specific health and wellness training programs to build key knowledge and skills are necessary	• This type of coaching provides content expertise to "coach the client to be a coach"

The vast majority of coaching is *transformational coaching*, and the requirements are threefold when it comes to the coach-client relationship. First, a "safe" environment in which the client can feel that he or she can discuss not only strengths to extend, but also areas for professional and personal development openly without fear of negative evaluation or backlash. Second, a clear understanding that the relationship is not one in which the coach has an evaluative or supervisory role over the client. Third, a detailed conversation and agreement is made among the client, coach, and sponsoring agency or supervisor/manager, if applicable, around the boundaries of confidentiality, including information received or given to the coach from individuals outside the coaching relationship. Once established, this agreement should be made in writing, with the appropriate signatures of the client, coach, and sponsoring agency designee or supervisor/manager.

Often, the feedback collected to develop improvement goals includes the following coaching tools:

- Self-assessments, surveys, and validated instruments
- Open-ended coaching assessment to discover areas for improvement
- Direct evaluation/feedback by a supervisor or designated workplace advisor
- Confidential 360-degree evaluations by supervisor(s), peers, direct reports, and other team members (facilitated by the coach or other designee)

There are multiple coaching assessments that are validated and commonly used by coaches to facilitate insight and to establish coaching goals. In best practice, a coach should choose the appropriate coaching assessment based on the needs of the client. Therefore, coaches, in addition to their certification status and experience, also should be selected based on their depth of training and certification in various coaching assessments. For example, the validated coaching assessments most commonly used (but not exhaustive) by these authors include those that evaluate key areas for leadership and workplace performance:

1. Emotional Intelligence (Eq-I 2.0)
2. Leadership (Hogan Leader Focus, DiSC Work of Leaders, CCL Compass)
3. 360 Evaluation (DiSC 363 for Leaders, Hogan 360, EQ 360, CCL Benchmarks)
4. Personality Tendencies (DiSC Workplace, Hogan Personality Inventory, Pearman Personality Indicator-a coachable adaptation of the Myers-Briggs Type Indicator)

Once clients gain clarity in understanding of the developmental area(s), coaches create motivation for change, breaking down the goals into smaller S.M.A.R.T. (Specific, Measurable, Achievable, Relevant, Timebound) goals. Once these goals are set, a learning plan is created to address the specified goals. The coach may be involved in some of the skills development areas, and often other mentors/experts are engaged to assist. The coach, however, is responsible for holding the client accountable for each goal, identifying successes as well as barriers to achieving the goals.

Transformational coaching has several subtypes: *performance coaching, career coaching, leadership coaching, business coaching, health and wellness coaching*. Of note, the American Medical Association recently published a handbook on medical education coaching that parallels the practice of transformational coaching.[14] The investigators define the practice of coaching medical education learners as *academic coaching*.[14] The handbook provides pragmatic practice guidelines to coaching and developing and evaluating a coaching program, which is still an emerging field in medicine.

Performance coaching, similar to clinical coaching, focuses on building a strong alliance and collecting feedback to improve the performance of the client. Crucial to the coaching relationship, the coaches are not involved in any way with, for example, the client's evaluation/grading system. Performance coaches provide insight to clients to discover their goals for improvement, and help clients improve their aptitude for life-long learning, so that they are better able to evaluate and self-monitor, and ask for help in general. Most often, a request for performance coaches is initiated by a supervisor or hiring organization to quickly address a performance gap in their employee.

Career coaching involves a creative, insight-oriented process that facilitates maximizing a client's personal and professional potential. Career coaches, through positive psychology and coaching principles, will open up a client's ability to understand the professional goals that they would like to achieve, elicit specific strategies and solutions, and hold the client responsible and accountable. This process helps clients create a more positive outlook on both work and life issues, while improving their leadership skills. Clients view career coaching as unlocking their potential to reconnect to their sense of purpose and passion or create new opportunities in their career development journey. A recent career coaching intervention in internal medicine interns has demonstrated efficacy in increasing resiliency and reducing burnout, and detailed information about how the internal coaching program was established is outlined.[11]

Leadership coaching targets not only existing leaders, but also clients who will be onboarding into a new leadership role, a potential talent who has been identified by their hiring organization. Leadership coaching includes topics covered by the ACHE mentioned previously. The coaches who practice leadership coaching often have current or prior experience in leadership roles or systems management.

Business coaching has a dual focus in helping the individual to have increased self-awareness and consider how to make changes in behavior or perspective that can help them as individuals and also the business in which they are employed. Business coaches also can provide relevant entrepreneurial or business expertise, often based on their own experience. A more extensive definition of business coaching by the WABC can be found at www.wabccoaches.com/includes/popups/definition.html.

Health and wellness coaching targets primarily patients, but occasionally includes coaching physicians and other health care providers on not only their own self-care strategies but also how to educate their patients. As population health and capitated contracts become more the norm, health and wellness coaching are being integrated into health and behavioral health organizations.

INTERNAL VERSUS EXTERNAL COACHING

Coaching interventions can be either internal or external. Internal coaches and their internal coaching programs are sponsored by the hiring organization, and the coaches are their employees. The benefits of an internal coach are that the coaches have experience and knowledge of the culture and politics of the system in which the client works. Internal coaches also have relationships with many of the human resources/faculty affairs leaders within the organizational structure, awareness of the unique issues in a strategic plan, and are better aligned not only with the client but also the organization. It is crucial that internal coaches clearly establish a confidentiality agreement that is strictly adhered to, despite the sponsor being the organization.

External coaches can be beneficial if there is concern about the client trusting the organization or his or her internal coach (ie, in performance coaching in which a clear issue must be addressed). Also, external coaches are used in leadership coaching, as they can provide specific expertise based on their own professional experience. In many organizations, a list of external coaches who have been vetted and cataloged for their expertise is maintained to ensure quality and "fit" of the coaches who have a better understanding of the systems and politics/cultural issues unique to their organization. External coaches must avoid the pitfall of aligning so strongly with the individual client that they become biased against an organization, which can prevent them from holding the client accountable for their intended goals.

GROUP AND TEAM-BASED GROUP COACHING

Group coaching can be a powerful type of coaching. Multiple clients who have common shared goals meet for regularly scheduled meetings facilitated by a coach. Similar to individual coaching, group coaching can include using coaching assessments, self-awareness, and other-awareness tools. On the other hand, the accountability is mainly derived from the peer group. Special attention should be placed on group adhesion/trust, shared understanding of communication outside of the group, and confidentiality.

Team-based group coaching can be helpful not only to newly formed teams, but also teams seeking to improve overall function and performance. In addition, specific coaching tools and assessments can address the group dynamics especially when working with a specific team. Lencioni and Okabayashi[15] have written about the 5 dysfunctions of a team that get in the way of achieving the results desired by a team, whereby one milestone must be achieved before addressing the next:

1. Absence of trust
2. Fear of conflict
3. Lack of commitment
4. Avoidance of accountability
5. Inattention to results

There are specific coaching tools that can address these dysfunctions and are best used in a team-based group-coaching format that focuses on delineating roles and responsibilities of each team member and aligning the team to common goals not only for the team but also alignment to the broader system or organization.

There are published reports of effective peer-mentoring groups in psychiatry that share similar elements of coaching.[16–20] The effectiveness included both benefits to the individual and to the sponsoring organization. The following common qualities led to successful outcomes: relationship between the peers and group facilitator, accountability, and shared group goals. In addition, groups that incorporate a participant to complete an individually mentored project, or "capstone project," during the course of their faculty development deepen the engagement to the group.[21] Group coaching can be a powerful intervention for special populations who may feel more comfortable with peers from a similar background: women,[16,17] minority,[18] trainees (such as residents, fellows, medical students),[19] and military[20] in psychiatry have been described in the literature. Furthermore, due to the use of a single coach facilitator with multiple clients in a group, the cost and return on investment may be greater for a sponsoring organization depending on the desired outcomes (engagement, retention, scholarly activity, academic promotions, succession planning). For example, recent review of faculty development programs underscores the need to integrate the shared goals of the sponsoring institution with the individual participant goals, as well as the importance of program evaluation to not only establish efficacy but also return on investment.[22]

INTEGRATING COACHING INTO ORGANIZATIONS AND PRACTICE

The University of Massachusetts Department of Psychiatry leadership (including the authors on this article) developed a Career Development and Research Office

(CDRO) to help the department create a culture of mentorship and develop a wide range of professional development programs and services to support individuals and teams throughout the department to improve their leadership, clinical, research, and teaching skills. (See Douglas Ziedonis and Mary S. Ahns' article, "Professional Development for Clinical Faculty in Academia: Focus on Teaching, Research and Leadership", in this issue). External coaches were hired in helping with individual leadership development and leadership team enhancement. These experiences were very positive and also led to the realization that there were not enough funds to solely hire external coaches and that an internal coaching program offering individual, leadership, peer, and team-based coaching could be developed. The authors sought their own coaching certification and integrated coaching into the culture of mentoring. Specific coaching services and activities were developed, targeting leadership, career development, performance skill development, and team building in a large department of more than 380 faculty members. Through developing a Leadership College, the CDRO provides group leadership coaching to interdisciplinary faculty and staff, which has led to increased emotional intelligence and leadership competencies.[23] Mindfulness training can help coaching skills and was integrated into several departmental programs. Coaching was particularly emphasized in a Mindful Physician Leadership Program in which enhancing mindfulness presence (eg, more aware of self and others, more focused, more compassionate to self and others) was foundational, and then mindful coaching skills were taught to help peer coaching using critical and simple coaching questions.[24–26]

SUMMARY

Ongoing professional development is essential for lifelong learning in psychiatry and all of health care across the career development lifespan. Coaching is emerging as an effective intervention to support career, personal, and leadership development of both individuals and teams in health care, given the high levels of volatility, uncertainty, and complexity that our physicians and organizations face. A coach, in contrast to a mentor, avoids giving direct advice to clients, while still providing self-awareness and other-awareness and accountability to their goals. Coaching can be practiced by existing mentors who develop skills in coaching, or by other practitioners depending on the desired outcomes. The use of coaches increases the flexibility of supporting our psychiatrists with a team of supporters, distilling the time of busy mentors to advise primarily on their content expertise.

REFERENCES

1. Johnson JE, Billingsley M, Crichlow T, et al. Professional development for nurses: mentoring along the U-shaped curve. Nurs Adm Q 2011;35(2):119–25.
2. ACHE Healthcare Executive (2019). Competencies Assessment Tool [pdf file]. Available at: https://www.ache.org/pdf/nonsecure/careers/competencies_booklet.pdf. Accessed June 8, 2019.
3. Adelman SA, Liebschutz JM. Coaching to enhance individual well-being, foster teamwork, and improve the health care system. N Engl J Med 2017.
4. McLean P. Completely revised handbook of coaching: a developmental approach. Hoboken (NJ): Wiley; 2012.
5. Institute of Coaching, McLean Hospital, Harvard Medical School Affiliate (2018). Becoming a coach. Available at: https://instituteofcoaching.org/coaching-overview/becoming-a-coach. Accessed June 8, 2019.

6. Sambunjak D, Straus SE, Marusić A. Mentoring in academic medicine: a systematic review. JAMA 2006;296(9):1103–15.

7. Meagher E, Taylor L, Probsfield J, et al. Evaluating research mentors working in the area of clinical translational science: a review of the literature. Clin Transl Sci 2011;4(5):353–8.

8. Glasgow ME, Weinstock B, Lachman V, et al. The benefits of a leadership program and executive coaching for new nursing academic administrators: one college's experience. J Prof Nurs 2009;25(4):204–10.

9. Thorn PM, Raj JM. A culture of coaching: achieving peak performance of individuals and teams in academic health centers. Acad Med 2012;87:1482–3.

10. Gifford KA, Fall LH. Doctor coach: a deliberate practice approach to teaching and learning clinical skills. Acad Med 2014;89:272–6.

11. Palamara K, Kauffman C, Stone VE, et al. Promoting success: a professional development coaching program for interns in medicine. J Grad Med Educ 2015;7:630–7.

12. Duan K, Sheu L. Behind closed doors. Med Teach 2017;39(5):558–9.

13. Sargeant J, Lockyer JM, Mann K, et al. The R2C2 model in residency education: how does it foster coaching and promote feedback use? Acad Med 2018;93(7): 1055–63.

14. Deiorio NM, Hammoud M, eds. Accelerating change in medical education coaching handbook. American Medical Association [pdf file]. Available at: https://www.ama-assn.org/education/coaching-medical-education-faculty-handbook. Accessed June 8, 2019.

15. Lencioni P, Okabayashi K. The five dysfunctions of a team. Hoboken (NJ): Wiley; 2012.

16. Lord JA, Mourtzanos E, McLaren K, et al. A peer mentoring group for junior clinician educators: four years' experience. Acad Med 2012;87(3):378–83.

17. Steiner JL, Mazure C, Siggins LD, et al. Teaching psychiatric residents about women and leadership. Acad Psychiatry 2004;28(3):243–6.

18. Yager J, Waitzkin H, Parker T, et al. Educating, training, and mentoring minority faculty and other trainees in mental health services research. Acad Psychiatry 2007;31(2):146–51.

19. Van Schalkwyk GI, Katz RB, Resignato J, et al. Effective research mentorship of residents: meeting the needs of early career physicians. Acad Psychiatry 2016; 41:326–32.

20. Warner CH, Bobo WV, Flynn J. Early career professional development issues for military academic psychiatrists. Acad Med 2005;29(5):437–42.

21. Mennin S, Kalishman S, Eklund MA, et al. Project-based faculty development by international health professions educators: practical strategies. Med tech 2013; 35:e971–7.

22. Gruppen LD. Faculty development in the health professions: a focus on research and practice, innovation and change in professional education. Berlin: Springer; 2014.

23. Ahn MS. Leadership agility training: building emotional intelligence through peer coaching. Podium Presentation presented at the Association of American Medical Colleges Group on Faculty Affairs Professional Development Conference. Vancouver, Canada, July 28, 2017.

24. Byron G, Ziedonis D, McGrath C, et al. Implementation of mindfulness training for mental health staff: organizational context and stakeholder perspectives. Mindfulness 2015;6(4):861–72.

25. Ziedonis D, Fulwiler C, Tonelli M. Integrating mindfulness into your daily routine. Vital Signs, a Publication of the Massachusetts Medical Society 2014;19(2):6.

26. Tonelli M, Fulwiler C, de Torrijos F, et al. Mindfulness in psychiatry program and emerging initiatives at the University of Massachusetts & UMass Memorial Health Care. Worcester Med 2016;80(2):14–5. Available at: http://www.wdms.org/PDF/0316WOMED.pdf.

Low-Resource Project-Based Interprofessional Development with Psychiatry Faculty

Erica Z. Shoemaker, MD, MPH[a],*, Myo Thwin Myint, MD[b],
Shashank V. Joshi, MD[c], Donald M. Hilty, MD, MBA[d,e]

KEYWORDS

- Faculty development • Professional development • Team-based • Project-based
- Interprofessional • Longitudinal • Mentorship

KEY POINTS

- Informal faculty development in groups can be conducted with minimal resources and yield both intangible (a sense of community and team skills) and tangible (scholarly papers and presentations) benefits.
- Small-scale projects done in interprofessional teams are helpful in building a positive work culture, socializing faculty, and emphasizing quality improvement, and may be the preferred option for junior faculty. Project-based faculty development done in the workplace and in an interprofessional group can benefit multiple parties: faculty, divisions, departments, medical schools, clinical affiliates, and academic medical centers.
- Project-based faculty development done in the workplace yields short-term wins and can change the long-term course of a faculty member's career.
- The combination of low costs, high yields, and improvements in team/interprofessional skills make project-based and peer-based learning feasible and sustainable in modern, resource-constrained medical schools and academic medical centers.

Disclosure Statement: The authors have nothing to disclose.
[a] Child and Adolescent Psychiatry, Keck School of Medicine, University of Southern California, LAC+ USC Medical Center, 2250 Alcazar Street, Suite 2200, Los Angeles, CA 90033, USA; [b] Triple Board & Child and Adolescent Psychiatry Programs, Tulane University School of Medicine, 1430 Tulane Avenue, #8055, New Orleans, LA 70112, USA; [c] Lucile Packard Children's Hospital @ Stanford, 401 Quarry Road, Stanford, CA 94305-5719, USA; [d] Mental Health, Northern California Veterans Administration Health Care System, 10535 Hospital Way, Mather, CA 95655 (116/SAC), USA; [e] Department of Psychiatry and Behavioral Sciences, UC Davis, Davis, CA, USA
* Corresponding author.
E-mail address: Erica.shoemaker@med.usc.edu

INTRODUCTION

In this article, the authors describe 4 faculty professional development projects. All 4 projects were based in the workplace and done in groups, and these groups were heterogeneous either by level of experience or by professional discipline. All 4 projects were inexpensive at startup, requiring mostly reallocated faculty and staff time as inputs. None of the projects were part of a formal professional development academy or classroom activity, yet all 4 projects yielded benefits in faculty morale and deepened interprofessional relationships. All 4 projects also enabled the participating faculty to have more tangible impact in their work as leaders, teachers, and scholars.

Formal faculty development can range from activities done solo (completing coursework for Continuing Medical Education or Maintenance of Certification credits), to those done 1:1 (such as an assigned mentor within an academic department to help with academic promotion), to work done as part of a classroom-based program (such as seminars on being a more effective teacher or on how to get work published). All of these activities may meet faculty members' needs for professional growth and generativity. These experiences can be a tool for improving faculty performance[1] and for recruiting, motivating, and retaining high-quality staff. This may be especially true for new and junior faculty, whereby the business literature has found that collaborative work with purpose may be among the best incentives to attract and retain young workers, rather than traditional incentives of money, titles, and long-term opportunities for investment.[2] Some of the most comprehensive faculty development programs include those described by Cornell University, the University of Toronto Center for Faculty Development, the Stanford Faculty Development Center, the Executive Leader in Academic Medicine (ELAM) program, and the Harvard Macy Program.[3–5]

These formal faculty development programs require some substantial investments, including time, meeting space, and other administrative supports. Time is also needed for faculty leader and presenter preparation (planning the curriculum) and presenter/attendee, and participation; opportunity costs include lost research or clinical revenue. Furthermore, because formal faculty development programs do not always produce immediately tangible results, or results that can be directly linked to the faculty development activity, it can be hard for departments and schools to justify the investment in these programs.[6–8] The combination of big investments up front and difficult-to-count outcomes can be an obstacle to a division or department trying to start a faculty development program. In contrast, the informal approaches described in this article are more feasible for resource-strapped divisions and busy faculty.

Whether done formally or informally, however, there is a growing consensus that faculty development done in groups, rather than 1:1, may be more successful.[3,9] Groups of 6 to 12 faculty members can form in a single worksite, a division, or from several departments around a common interest. Peer mentoring groups provide "faculty members with entry into a new intellectual and social community of like-minded individuals."[8] These groups can serve as a place for faculty to seek advice, find collaborators and role models, and find accountability for deadlines. As the group matures, it may coalesce into a "community of practice," where members form a community in which they are bonded by a shared purpose, a history of shared accomplishments, and emotional connections.[8,10] When group members are from different institutions or departments, "such communities often help participants overcome feelings of isolation in their own departments and divisions."[8] Although this intangible sense of community may seem like a "nice to have," Gast and colleagues[1] even noted that the subjective feeling of community in such a group is predictive of the tangible productivity of such groups.

This article focuses on faculty development projects that are affordable, feasible, and sustainable within the modern, resource-constrained, academic medical center. It is our thesis that faculty development that is informal, done in an interprofessional group, and is project-based is best able to leverage existing resources in the workplace. Furthermore, such activities can yield products that benefit the participants, their departments, and their medical center in both tangible and intangible ways and in both the short-term and long-term. For the 4 case examples, the authors describe the project and its goal, the team members, the required inputs, and the outputs/benefits that grew from the project.

INFORMAL FACULTY DEVELOPMENT IN GROUPS CAN BE CONDUCTED WITH MINIMAL RESOURCES YET YIELD BOTH TANGIBLE AND INTANGIBLE BENEFITS

Faculty, training directors, and department chairs need approaches, skills, and knowledge to promote academic scholarship within their divisions and departments. Directors of residency and fellowship training, in particular, may be starting off in their leadership role early in their career, before they have mature scholarship skills. Early career faculty may be seeking a forum for sage, unbiased, and confidential advice on challenges in their educational leadership role, especially from those not directly within their department. In addition, those same training directors may find it challenging to find time to complete scholarly work, given multiple competing demands, especially clinical productivity. Some fortunate faculty find a mentor, have a peer mentoring group, or work productively in a solo manner in their home department.[11] Yet many have the ambition to be academically productive but are not progressing.[12]

One way to meet this unmet need for a learning community of psychiatry faculty is through videoconferencing technology. The same technology being used for telemedicine clinical services can be harnessed to team-based or peer-based learning.[13] Synchronous (video) telepsychiatry leverages care for diagnosis/assessment, consultation, and a range of treatments in many populations (eg, adult, child, geriatric), settings and cultures with outcomes are comparable to in-person care.[14,15] Now, e-models of care based on telephone and e-mail curbside consultations improve clinical, educational, administration and other types of outcomes.[16] Telehealth distance mentoring is used for students,[17] surgical fellows,[18] perioperative education,[19] and health researchers.[20] Distance mentoring is also an element of top-flight professional development programs like ELAM or the Harvard Macy Fellowship.[4] Peer mentoring groups done at a distance provide some advantages over in-person groups: it allows members to benefit from the experience and knowledge of faculty at a different site, it allows a higher standard of confidentiality, and it allows for customization of shared interests that may not be available to faculty at their home institution. Of note, peer mentoring groups done via videoconferencing do require a skillful facilitator and highly motivated faculty.

Case 1: Child and Adolescent Psychiatry Tele-Writing Group

The Project and the Goal: In 2014, the team facilitator (DH) and cofounder (SVJ) began a discussion about the difficulty that child and adolescent psychiatry (CAP) training directors and faculty have in generating scholarly work that disseminates their knowledge and helps them progress in their careers. They identified that obstacles to scholarly productivity included not only competing demands from the faculty's training and clinical roles but also difficulty finding collaborators and mentors in their home institutions and national organizations. They surmised that a simple monthly teleconference could provide peer support and supervision and also structure and motivation for producing scholarly projects. A separate discussion at the American College of Psychiatry (DH and a future member of the group) tilted the focus toward CAP.

This pilot project is a monthly, 1-hour videoconference or teleconference call that began in summer 2015 and continues to the present. The call is split with half of time used for member check-ins and the other half used for discussions of writing group projects. Like any new group, matters such as confidentiality and attendance required for participation were agreed on at the beginning. There was often substantial overlap between topics at check-ins (faculty challenged by working with trainees of a different generation, technology in clinical care and education) and agreed-on writing projects. These calls were supplemented by in-person meet-ups at national meetings once per year. Between meetings, participants were expected to be progressing on writing projects and submissions to conferences on their own time; much of this correspondence was done via e-mail.

Team:

- Team facilitator: advanced career psychiatrist and scholar with extensive experience in faculty development, telehealth, and distance mentoring
- Nine team members: all child and adolescent psychiatrists involved in medical education, ranging from early career faculty immediately out of fellowship to full professors

Resources:

- Teleconference and videoconference line
- Facilitator skill in distance mentoring and leading heterogeneous groups to produce scholarly work
- Highly motivated faculty
- Faculty time, facilitator: Web-based videoconference set-up, e-mailing follow-up for meetings, networking, recruiting new members, 2 to 4 hours of individual mentoring, writing time (monthly)
- Faculty time, members: 1-hour video call or teleconference, intermittent e-mail correspondence, variable time writing/preparing presentations (monthly)

Outcomes and Benefits in Faculty Development (over 3 years):

- 6 publications/articles in press (including 3 articles in this issue of *Psychiatric Clinics of North America*)
- 2 manuscripts submitted/in preparation
- 8 presentations at national meetings
- Increased self-efficacy and confidence among members in their leadership role
- Reduced feelings of isolation or anxiety among members in their roles in their home institutions
- Academic promotion and national leadership opportunities for members

Key Concepts for Formal Faculty Development:

- Peer mentoring, writing groups, networking

Key References:

- Brandon C, Jamadar D, Girish G, Dong Q, Morag Y, Mullan P. Peer support of a faculty "writer's circle" increases confidence and productivity in generating scholarship. Acad Radiol. 2015;22:534–8.
- Schubert A. Tele-conferencing, distance learning and tele-mentoring: New technology harnessed for perioperative education. J Educ Perioper Med. 2000;2(1):E012.

PROJECT-BASED FACULTY DEVELOPMENT DONE IN THE WORKPLACE IN AN INTERPROFESSIONAL GROUP CAN BENEFIT FACULTY, MEDICAL SCHOOLS, AND ACADEMIC MEDICAL CENTERS

Most psychiatrists desire for their work to be impactful in their real-world workplaces: medical schools and academic medical centers. Work that is sequestered in the classroom is less able to make change in medical education and clinical care. Classroom work is limited by the fact that it may be unable to generate buy-in (and resources) from leadership/administration.[21] This is especially true for projects with goals that are primarily educational improvement; a goal that is not always the highest priority for administrators.[1,21] To garner support in their workplaces, faculty will need to appreciate the diverse needs of their workplaces: financial, regulatory, even prestige/reputation. By considering these diverse needs, and planning projects that meet the needs of their workplace as well as their own need for development, faculty can begin to generate institutional buy-in and garner institutional resources (money, administrative support) to create and implement impactful projects.

However, when faculty undertake these real-world projects, they are likely to run into obstacles. The first obstacle is that they are probably unable to complete a project individually; there is simply too much work. The second obstacle is that they probably are not knowledgeable about every process or piece of work that needs to be done. This is where faculty recruiting a truly interprofessional team becomes essential. With practice, the workplace team may bring nurses, therapists, and hospital administrators/business managers into the learning community. All members can make substantial contributions to quality and feel trusted and take ownership of the results of team efforts.[22]

Health care organizations are currently emphasizing quality and performance improvement. Quality improvement (QI) is a need partly because of regulatory pressure but also because, in business terms, quality is the most significant determinant in the long-run success or failure of any organization, even more than cost and productivity.[2] QI methodology, inherently based on small and iterative process changes, also emphasizes formation of a diverse team for implementing projects. Indeed, the goal is creating a culture to look at problems without blame or shame and to foster input, teamwork, and collaboration.

Case 2: Implementation of Sensory Modalities for Reducing Aggression, Seclusion, and Restraint on an Adolescent Inpatient Psychiatric Ward

The Project and The Goal: A 10-bed adolescent inpatient ward experienced acute increases in aggressive behaviors by patients on the ward, with a parallel rise in seclusion and restraint episodes. This increase coincided with a change in the patient population to include more adolescents with intellectual disability and autism spectrum disorder. Traditional psychiatric methods, reevaluation of diagnosis and medication, increased nursing supervision, psychotherapy groups, and behavior plans, were proving impractical or ineffective at reducing aggressive behaviors and episodes of seclusion and restraint.

The CAP division chief (author ES) called a series of meetings with ward staff and began e-mail and phone discussions about responses to this problem. A newly hired occupational therapist with experience using sensory modalities (weighted vest and lap-pads, plastic tube "snake" that is worn around the neck) suggested implementing such methods as part of regular ward programming. ES and leadership in occupational therapy (OT) threw their support behind this change, and the occupational therapist began the process of ordering sensory modalities and planning implementation. This programming is now offered to all patients on the ward for 1 hour on all weekdays. The occupational therapist invites nursing assistants assigned to monitor patients to themselves use the noodles or weighted vests during the OT hour.

This change in programming became the focus of a QI project and a symbol of the new team culture. This project was planned and conducted by the occupational therapist and the advisor for QI for the department. The outcomes of this study were remarkable: in the classroom/schooling hour following OT programming on the ward, the average number of "acting out" episodes decreased from more than 14 to fewer than 2. Nursing staff also reported a subjective improvement in their sense of calm and well-being. Interprofessional staff most likely felt more "part of" the department, as their work was the essential ingredient in making the ward safer.

The Team:

- Occupational therapist
- OT supervisor
- Nursing assistants
- CAP chief (author ES)
- QI advisor

Resources:

- Occupational therapist with training and experience in sensory modalities
- Instigation and moral support by OT and child psychiatry leadership
- Purchase of sensory equipment (from existing OT budget)
- OT and QI Director time planning intervention and measurement and preparing reports
- OT and nursing time implementing the project (no extra hours of staff time)

Outcomes:

- Improved safety of patients
- Improved safety of nursing staff
- Education for nursing and psychiatry staff and about the utility of these methods
- OT staff presented at Institute for Healthcare Improvement Scientific Symposium in 2018
- Recognition for this achievement within the medical center; prestige for the OT and the Department Psychiatry and Behavioral Sciences

Benefits for Faculty Development:

- Child Psychiatry Service Chief gained experience as a facilitator and supporter, rather than leader, of change

Key Concepts for Formal Faculty Development:

- QI, Interprofessional Teams

Key Reference:

- Tess A, Vidyarthi A, Yang J, Myers JS. Bridging the Gap: A framework and strategies for integrating the quality and safety mission of teaching hospitals and graduate medical education. Acad Med. 2015; 90:1251–7.

Case 3: Starting Up Integrated Care at a Federally Qualified Health Center

The Project and The Goal: A federally qualified health center (FQHC) was using a traditional screen-and-refer model for mental health services within their clinic. In this model, a pediatric provider would identify children and families with mental health needs and then refer them to a triple-board child psychiatrist and a therapist for specialty mental health services within the clinic. These specialty mental health services were provided by author MTM (0.2 full-time equivalent [FTE]) and a full-time therapist. As has been described in many systems, this process was leading to delays in children and families receiving mental health care and frustration/stress among pediatric medical providers. The clinic implemented 2 changes to speed children and families to care. The first intervention was to hire integrated care social workers trained to work in the integrated model, one of whose time is included in seeing pediatric patients (0.2 FTE). This new social worker provided service both in the integrated and specialty mental health model. The child psychiatrist and original therapist continued to provide specialty-level mental health care.

The second intervention was to reallocate some administrative time of members of the interprofessional team to biweekly huddles. These huddles are held in high importance in the clinic, and they are attended by an interprofessional team ranging from the medical case workers to the child psychiatrist. These huddles serve multiple purposes. First, these huddles matched families' needs to the correct level of mental health care and ensured that families who needed care actually got linked to the integrated or specialty mental health teams. Second, the interaction in these huddles shared knowledge and developed skills in all team members, such as helping pediatric providers learn how to motivate reluctant families to engage in mental health treatment, building mental health providers' knowledge of the impact of physical health conditions (such as human immunodeficiency virus) on mental health, increasing pediatric providers' comfort in providing some psychotropic and parent counseling about mental health issues in their pediatric visits, and improving the medical and nursing care providers' knowledge of social interventions to help families (housing and transportation assistance). Last, inviting pediatric and psychiatric residents has improved the next generation's knowledge and attitude toward integrated care.

The Team:

- Pediatricians

- Triple-board psychiatrist (author MTM)

- Rotating residents and medical students

- Integrated care social workers (ICSWs)

- Case managers

- Nurse practitioners

- Nurses

Resources:

- 0.2 FTE of ICSW time

- Reallocation of protected administrative time of multiple team members: existing resource

Outcomes:

- Reduced waiting times for patients accessing mental health care

- Reduced stress and improved satisfaction among pediatric providers

- Improved knowledge, attitudes, and skills among all team members

- Team cohesion and sense of community among interprofessional team

Benefits for Faculty Development:

- Improved consultation skills on the part of triple-board child psychiatrist

- Offer from leadership to pay for more child psychiatry time (potential for increased faculty salary support in the future)

Key Concepts for Formal Faculty Development:

- Mission-based budgeting, effective meetings, capacity building

Key Reference:

- SAMHSA HRSA Center for Integrated Health Solutions. Primary and Behavioral Health Integration; Guiding Principles for Workforce Development. Available at: https://www. integration.samhsa.gov/about-us/about-cihs. Accessed April 25, 2019.

PROJECT-BASED PROFESSIONAL DEVELOPMENT DONE IN THE WORKPLACE YIELDS SHORT-TERM WINS THAT CAN BE LEVERAGED TO CHANGE THE LONG-TERM COURSE OF A FACULTY MEMBER'S CAREER

The previous section discussed workplace-based projects that have been relatively short-term, implemented over 2 to 3 years. In this section, we describe a project that has been built over a 15-year period. This project illustrates the power for steadily growing impact over that time.[23,24] In addition, the interprofessional nature of this project has allowed the child and adolescent psychiatrist and CAP trainees to gain experience with being one member of a team centered around a student, rather than solely being the provider directing treatment decisions.

Case 4: A University-Schools Partnership Aimed at Residency Training, School Mental Health, and Interprofessional Collaboration

The Project and The Goal: A charter high school struggled with how best to integrate the mental health and educational needs of its students, and of how to promote compassion, satisfaction, and self-efficacy of its teachers and staff. Before this project, the school was using community providers who would come to the site weekly and provide direct mental health services to students. This process leads to students being "served" with regard to their mental health needs, but educators often felt uninformed regarding students' mental health and treatment. This led to frustration in both administrators and teachers, as they received little to no information regarding a student's therapeutic progress due to what they perceived as "the Great Wall of HIPAA [Health Insurance Portability and Accountability Act]."

Two weekly interprofessional team meetings were begun. The first was a meeting of front-line education and mental health staff, forming a team of informed and trusted adults around each student. The second meeting is a leadership meeting involving the child and adolescent psychiatrist, the manager of student services, psychologist supervisor, and lead guidance counselor. These meetings served as a mechanism for education, team-building, and spreading best practices for self-care (and burnout prevention) among all members, and the data collected informed future improvements.

This intervention started small but has resulted in gradually building resources and commitment from both the university and the school district. Even when FTE streams were reduced (temporarily), the school worked with a foundation to support a small amount of the faculty member's time. This commitment from the school and engagement with the faculty changed this faculty member's career trajectory, via immersion into clinical, scholarly, and policy projects with members of the school leadership. Trainees have benefited, not only in the school as a training site, but from a new perspective as part of a team. The experience became more student-centered rather than doctor-centered, so they could better appreciate the important and central roles of others on a team and leverage their credentials to advocate on behalf of a particular student or program. The "lived example" of this project as community-based research and interprofessional education has been so persuasive that other schools within the university and other school districts have been drawn to participate.

The Team:

- Child and adolescent psychiatrist (author SVJ)
- Supervising psychologist
- Graduate students in psychology
- CAP fellow
- Lead guidance counselor
- Manager of Student Services (who serves as case manager as well)
- Leadership: Principal, dean of students, lead teacher advisor for selected students

Resources:

- Protected time for the team (reallocation of administrative time to help make clinical time more efficient)
- 1 FTE, manager of student services (school district employee)
- 8 hours per week, 0.2 FTE child psychologist (paid for by school)
- 2 hours per week, 0.05 FTE child and adolescent psychiatrist (paid for by hospital grant in community engagement)
- 20 hours per week, total commitment from graduate students in psychology (practicum experience, hence no cost to school)

Outcomes (over 15 years):

- Improved student mental health care (outcomes evaluations at site)
- Expansion of clinical model to include visits in their home and in the community, addiction prevention
- Later school start times
- Collaboration with additional school districts
- Improved trainee and faculty satisfaction and well-being (measured on burnout/compassion survey annually)
- Training experience of a CAP fellow and several psychology trainees annually

Benefits for Faculty Development (over 15 years):

- Several academic publications
- 2 policy statements on suicide prevention
- Author SVJ with substantive body of accomplishment as a school psychiatrist

Key Concepts for Formal Faculty Development:

- Consolidating gains, building on small wins to produce more change, breaking down silos

Key Reference:

- Kotter J. *Leading Change.* Boston, MA: Harvard Business Review Press; 2012. P. 137–151.

DISCUSSION

The authors presented 4 examples of project-based faculty development ranging from small and simple (a teleconference-based peer writing group), to projects done in small interprofessional work units (implementing sensory modalities on an inpatient ward, starting up an integrated care intervention at an FQHC), to a multistage project that spanned a decade and led to grants and programs that extended care to a new group of patients, trained many classes of child psychiatry fellows, and changed the trajectory of a career (school mental health).

All 4 of these projects yielded subjective improvements of being part of a community of professionals. Although this subjective sense may seem a "nice but not necessary" element of the modern academic medicine workplace, many have wondered[21,25] if this subjective sense of community may help prevent burnout and attrition among faculty and health care providers. Furthermore, as Steinert[7] noted in the 2017 review of faculty development, "supportive relationships with colleagues, noted in over 30% of the studies, appeared to enable the accomplishment of shared goals and individual success." The support of a team or professional community may be both nice and necessary for team success. In addition, as health care requires interprofessional teams to achieve optimal outcomes and reasonable costs, the collaborative interprofessional skills built in these projects may be a major element of success for members[22].

Projects implemented in the workplace have 2 advantages that help them make a large impact when compared with classroom-based work. Workplace-based projects that serve multiple needs of the medical center/medical school can attract more resources—resources of faculty and staff knowledge and skills, access to budgets that can be repurposed, and dedicated faculty and staff time—than classroom-based projects. Inevitably, projects working with more resources have the potential to become impactful. Last, workplace-based projects that are small yet successful can continue to attract resources over time, leading to longitudinal gains and larger magnitude of gains.

There are limitations of such informal, workplace-based projects. Previous reviews have found that faculty development activities that are not accompanied by "grounding" coursework are often ineffective.[8,9] All of the authors have participated in substantial formal and classroom-based faculty development, including medical education fellowships, leadership academies, and even master's degree programs. Although the work described in this article was not part of a classroom assignment, the authors were using knowledge and skills they obtained through previous formal education. Next, success of interventions is usually measured in quantitative terms, which most of the projects have to a degree, but not just in terms of publications and grants. Mentoring, though, meets tangible and intangible needs.[25] Last, we must acknowledge that this article is a report of the personal experience of the authors; none of the projects described have undergone prospective, rigorous evaluation as suggested by leaders in the field of faculty development.[7] Like patient-centered clinical care, effective rather than efficacious interventions may be so customized to the local team and workplace that they may not lend themselves to controlled scientific evaluation. Nevertheless, the narratives and their benefits appear substantial and contain elements generalizable to faculty development programs at other institutions.

REFERENCES

1. Gast I, Schildkamp K, van der Veen JT. Team-based professional development interventions in higher education: a systematic review. Rev Educ Res 2017; 87(4):736–67.
2. Rateri S, Evans JR. Principles of operations management. Mason (OH): Thomas Southwestern; 2005. p. 163–95.
3. Pololi LH, Evans AT. Group peer mentoring: an answer to the faculty mentoring problem? A successful program at a large academic department of medicine. J Contin Educ Health Prof 2015;35(3):192–200.
4. Helitzer DL, Newbill SL, Morahan PS, et al. Perceptions of skill development of participants in three national career development programs for women faculty in academic medicine. Acad Med 2014;89(6):896–903.
5. Johansson J, Skeff K, Stratos G. Clinical teaching improvement: the transportability of the Stanford Faculty Development Program. Med Teach 2009;31(8): e377–82.
6. Steinert Y, Mann K, Anderson B, et al. A systematic review of faculty development initiatives designed to enhance teaching effectiveness: a 10-year update. BEME Guide No. 40. Med Teach 2016;38(8):769–86.
7. Steinert Y. Faculty development: from program design and implementation to scholarship. GMS J Med Educ 2017;34(4):Doc49.

8. O'Sullivan PS, Irby DM. Reframing research on faculty development. Acad Med 2011;86(4):421–8.
9. Lord J, Mourtzanos E, McLaren K, et al. A peer mentoring group for junior clinician educators: four years' experience. Acad Med 2012;87(3):378–83.
10. Macmillan DW, Chavis DM. Sense of community: a definition and theory. J Community Psychol 1986;14:6–23.
11. Brandon C, Jamadar D, Girish G, et al. Peer support of a faculty "writer's circle" increases confidence and productivity in generating scholarship. Acad Radiol 2015;22:534–8.
12. Landsberger SA, Scott EL, Hulvershorn LA, et al. Mentorship of clinical-track junior faculty: impact of a facilitated peer-mentoring program to promote scholarly productivity. Acad Psychiatry 2013;37(4):288–9.
13. Wakefield DS, Kienzle MG, Zollo SA, et al. Health care providers' perceptions of telemedicine services. Telemed J 1997;3(1):59–65.
14. Hilty DM, Yellowlees PM, Nesbitt TS. Evolution of telepsychiatry to rural sites: change over time in types of referral and PCP knowledge, skill, and satisfaction. Gen Hosp Psychiatry 2006;28(5):367–73.
15. Hilty DM, Ferrer D, Parish MB, et al. The effectiveness of telemental health: a 2013 review. Telemed J E Health 2013;19(6):444–54.
16. Hilty DM, Rabinowitz TR, McCarron RM, et al. An update on telepsychiatry and how it can leverage collaborative, stepped, and integrated services to primary care. Psychosomatics 2018;59(3):227–50.
17. Loera JA, Kuo YF, Rahr RR. Telehealth distance mentoring of students. Telemed J E Health 2007;13(1):45–50.
18. Falcone JL, Croteau AJ, Schenarts KD. The role of gender and distance mentoring in the surgical education research fellowship. J Surg Educ 2015;72(2):330–7.
19. Schubert A. Tele-conferencing, distance learning and tele-mentoring: new technology harnessed for perioperative education. J Educ Perioper Med 2000;2(1): E012.
20. Xu X, Schneider M, DeSorbo-Quinn AL, et al. Distance mentoring of health researchers: three case studies across the career-development trajectory. Health Psychol Open 2017;4(2). 2055102917734388.
21. Mennin S, Kalishman S, Eklund MA, et al. Project-based faculty development by international health professions educators: practical strategies. Med Teach 2013; 35(2):e971–7.
22. Tess A, Vidyarthi A, Yang J, et al. Bridging the gap: a framework and strategies for integrating the quality and safety mission of teaching hospitals and graduate medical education. Acad Med 2015;90:1251–7.
23. SAMHSA HRSA Center for Integrated Health Solutions. Primary and behavioral health integration; guiding principles for workforce development. Available at: https://www.integration.samhsa.gov/about-us/about-cihs. Accessed April 25, 2019.
24. Kotter J. Leading change. Boston (MA): United States of America: Harvard Business Review Press; 2012. p. 137–51.
25. Shollen SL, Bland CJ, Center BA, et al. Relating mentor type and mentoring behaviors to academic medicine faculty satisfaction and productivity at one medical school. Acad Med 2014;89:1267–75.

Lifelong Learning for Professional Development in Psychiatry
Pedagogy, Innovations, and Maintenance of Certification

Jeffrey Hunt, MD[a],*, Elizabeth Brannan, MD[b], Sandra Sexson, MD[c]

KEYWORDS

- Lifelong learning • Continuing professional development
- Maintenance of certification • Adult learning theory

KEY POINTS

- Model programs in lifelong learning should be designed based on principles of adult learning theory.
- Model programs should tap into the metacognitive processes involved in creating durable knowledge and skills.
- Passive types of continuing medical education and unguided self-assessment have been shown to be ineffective.
- The American Board of Psychiatry and Neurology Maintenance of Certification Pilot Project uses educational techniques that increase the promotion of both durable and efficient learning.
- Lifelong learning within the context of maintenance of certification programs will benefit from the innovations emerging from medical education research using technology and assessments strategies.

Disclosure Statement: Dr J. Hunt receives honoraria from John Wiley Publishers. Drs E. Brannan and S. Sexson report no conflicts related to this article.

[a] Child and Adolescent Psychiatry Fellowship and Triple Board Program, Division of Child and Adolescent Psychiatry, Alpert Medical School of Brown University, Bradley Hospital, 1011 Veterans Memorial Parkway, East Providence, RI 02915, USA; [b] Division of Child and Adolescent Psychiatry, Alpert Medical School of Brown University, Bradley Hospital, 1011 Veterans Memorial Parkway, East Providence, RI 02915, USA; [c] Child, Adolescent and Family Psychiatry, CAP Residency Training, Department of Psychiatry and Health Behavior, Medical College of Georgia at Augusta University, 997 St. Sebastian Way, Augusta, GA 30912, USA
* Corresponding author.
E-mail address: Jeffrey_hunt@brown.edu

Psychiatr Clin N Am 42 (2019) 425–437
https://doi.org/10.1016/j.psc.2019.05.014
0193-953X/19/© 2019 Elsevier Inc. All rights reserved.

Abbreviations	
ABMS	American Board of Medical Specialties
ABPN	American Board of Psychiatry and Neurology
APA	American Psychiatric Association
CME	Continuing medical education
CPD	Continuing professional development
MOC	Maintenance of certification
PIP	Performance in practice
RMF	Retrieval–monitoring–feedback
SA	Self-assessment

INTRODUCTION

Substantial inconsistencies in the delivery of quality evidenced based health care in the United States have been reported, indicating that 30% to 40% of patients do not receive evidence-based care and that 25% of the care delivered is not needed or actually harmful to patients.[1] This crisis has led to an increased demand for greater physician accountability, improved patient safety, and better quality of care.[2,3] Improved continued education for physicians has been considered to be an important part of the response to these challenges. The goal of continuing professional development (CPD) or lifelong learning is to ensure that physicians possess the required knowledge, skill, attitudes, and abilities to maintain and enhance competence and improve performance within their professional roles. However, studies of the effectiveness of formal CPD in enhancing competence and performance suggest that a substantial gap persists between the evidence available to inform practice and its translation into improved quality of care.[4–6]

The American Board of Medical Specialties (ABMS) which includes the American Board of Psychiatry and Neurology (ABPN) and the Accreditation Council for Continuing Medical Education and its member organizations promote standards that focus on changes in physicians' medical knowledge, skills, or abilities; actual performance on the job; and patient outcomes.[7] However, it remains unclear how best to conduct continuing medical education (CME) so as to positively affect the health of patients and the public. Traditional CME has been a time-based system of credits awarded for attending conferences, workshops, or lectures. The activities are typically teacher initiated, using passive educational models (eg, lecture) despite evidence that more active and individually reflective educational processes benefit physician learning.[8] Published work also indicates that CME, no matter how well-planned, often cannot produce changes in physician performance and patient health status by itself.[9]

The authors describe the literature concerning lifelong learning in medicine. They then review the history and current status of the ABPN Maintenance of Certification (MOC) program as an example of a model of lifelong learning and CPD. The final sections include a discussion of new innovations to consider in CPD and a reflection about the state of lifelong learning within the context of psychiatry MOC.

MODEL PROGRAMS SHOULD BE DESIGNED BASED ON PRINCIPLES OF ADULT LEARNING THEORY

Some medical education research over the past 20 years has demonstrated the effectiveness of CME in enhancing learning, if it is planned and implemented according to approaches that have been shown to work.[10,11] A recent expert consensus forum reviewed the evidence relating to how physicians learn and they proposed core principles from that research that should be used to plan formal educational activities designed to facilitate physician life long learning.[12] These include (1) recognizing an opportunity for learning, (2) searching for resources for learning, (3) engaging in learning to address an opportunity for improvement, (4) trying out what was learned, and (5) incorporating what was learned in new situations. These principles are very similar to those promoted by Kolb[13] and Armstrong and Parsa Parsi.[14] The experiential learning theory has merit regarding the mechanisms of self-directed learning. It was thought that self-directed learners would tend to be assimilators and reflectors and therefore to support learners in becoming more self-directed, they should be encouraged to adopt a more reflective learning style.[15] Interestingly, this turned out not to be the case; a study by Brookfield[16] found that successful self-directed adult learners were more likely to be activist—accommodators not reflector—assimilators. The willingness to network to problem solve led to more durable learning for the activist-accommodators, whereas the more autonomous reflectors kept themselves to themselves and sought less help. The key determinants of self-direction might not be learning style or personality type, but the metacognitive processes that determine both according to some medical education researchers.[17] A recent systematic review by the Cochrane Collaboration concluded that workshops using interactive formats could lead to moderately large changes in physician practice.[18,19]

The most effective CPD programs to foster lifelong learning would be designed and implemented with the principles of andragogy, the art and science of helping adults learn, as their guide (**Box 1**).

These principles fit with the trajectory of psychiatric medical education and practice. By the time psychiatrists have completed medical school, residency, and possibly a fellowship, they are in the phase of being able to direct their own learning and draw on increasingly abundant clinical and life experiences. If the educational material is relevant, the motivation is there. To be relevant, programs need to understand what the learners already know and what they need, and want, to know. Learners also need to understand the criteria for success before undertaking the learning task, and this will lead to more goal-directed behaviors (**Box 2**).

Programs also need to be mindful that individuals have different primary learning styles, the 3 major styles being visual, auditory, and kinesthetic (https://online.rutgers.edu/blog/principles-of-adult-learning-theory).[20]

Box 1
Assumptions about adult learners

Malcolm Knowles, who developed the principles of andragogy in the 1980s, proposed that adult learners:
- Move from dependency to increasing self-directedness as they mature and can direct their own learning
- Draw on their accumulated reservoirs of life experiences to aid learning
- Are ready to learn when assuming new social or life roles
- Are problem centered and want to apply new learning immediately
- Are motivated to learn by internal rather than external factors

Adapted from the Literacy Information and Communication System (LINCS). TEAL Center Fact Sheet No. 11: Adult Learning Theories. Available at: https://lincs.ed.gov/state-resources/federal-initiatives/teal/guide/adultlearning. Accessed May 8 2019; with permission.

Box 2
Implications for practice

Malcolm Knowles proposed that educators and educational programs for adult learners should consider the following:
- Set a cooperative climate for learning
- Assess the learners' specific needs and interests
- Develop learning objectives based on the learners' needs, interests, and skill levels
- Design sequential activities to achieve the objectives
- Work collaboratively with the learner to select methods, materials, and resources for instruction
- Evaluate the quality of the learning experience and make adjustment, as needed, while assessing needs for further learning

Adapted from the Literacy Information and Communication System (LINCS). TEAL Center Fact Sheet No. 11: Adult Learning Theories. Available at: https://lincs.ed.gov/state-resources/federal-initiatives/teal/guide/adultlearning. Accessed May 8 2019; with permission.

A related and important point about problem- or project-based learning is that it needs to be balanced with the fact that learners need sufficient content knowledge to make connections. A recent review article[21] indicated that problem-based methods of teaching and learning are most effective only after learners have attained sufficient surface knowledge and are now working for deeper knowledge and skill. This finding applies to CPD, at which stage learners' knowledge is fuller but process and skill are still evolving. This finding also applies to CPD in that if a novel treatment modality comes out, psychiatrists who completed training years ago may need to learn about it in a different way (eg, direct teaching for knowledge before any skills-based work) than psychiatrists who completed training more recently and already had some exposure and basic knowledge development and now need to hone the skill/process.

MODEL PROGRAMS SHOULD TAP INTO THE METACOGNITIVE PROCESSES INVOLVED IN CREATING DURABLE KNOWLEDGE AND SKILLS

No matter how effective a CPD program is in solidifying and expanding psychiatric knowledge and skills at the time of learning, patients, regulatory boards, and learners themselves care most about how durable this learning will be and how able learners will be to translate it to their actual practice. Rawson and Dunlosky[22] (2013) discuss the retrieval–monitoring–feedback (RMF) technique, which is a "learning technology to promote both durable and efficient student learning of key concepts from course material" and could be adapted for CME and to foster lifelong learning.

There are 3 steps in the RMF technique:

Step 1: Key concepts are presented for initial study
Step 2: RMF trials
- Phase 1 of each trial: retrieval practice = the concept term is presented as a cue and the learner attempts to type the correct definition into the computer
- Phase 2 of each trial: monitoring = the learner monitors the quality of the retrieved response using computer-generated feedback, and the learner evaluates whether their response includes the key concepts
- Phase 3 of each trial: feedback = the correct answer is presented intact for a self-paced restudy opportunity

Step 3: Scheduling retrieval practice
- The RMF technique uses learners' monitoring judgments to schedule practice of concepts in a manner that will lead to durable retention, because we know that spaced retrieval practice effects generalize to more complex material

What, then, is the optimal schedule of retrieval practice? Knowing this could help CME programs better effect durable change in practice based on knowledge and skill acquired in the initial program. Rawson and Dunlosky[23] (2011) studied this question for RMF and reported that,

> *A consistent qualitative pattern emerged: The effects of initial learning criterion and relearning were sub additive, such that the effects of initial learning criterion were strong prior to relearning but then diminished as relearning increased. Relearning had pronounced effects on long-term retention with a relatively minimal cost in terms of additional practice trials. On the basis of the overall patterns of durability and efficiency, our prescriptive conclusion for students is to practice recalling concepts to an initial criterion of 3 correct recalls and then to relearn them 3 times at widely spaced intervals.*

Although this concept applies directly only to the RMF technique, we can use such studies to understand the relevant metacognitive processes involved in durable knowledge and skill acquisition and as a jumping off point for more effective CPD program development. CME for content/knowledge could be designed with these concepts in mind to help assess and maintain current knowledge and practice rather than every-10-year computer-based multiple-choice tests. The use of smart phones, online group forums, apps that supply manageable chunks of assessment questions, and other technologies that allow efficient, electronic assessments that learners can access independently at spaced intervals could facilitate this process.

For optimal effectiveness, the assessment and monitoring approach should match the concept being taught. Programs should keep in mind that RMF and other similar assessment and monitoring techniques would then be more relevant to content/knowledge learning than to skill development, professionalism, communication, or quality improvement, which are equally important parts of CPD. It would be reasonable to consider, however, that for skill-based or professionalism and communication-based CME, simulation sessions, peer review of actual practice, or problem-based learning could be done initially to a predefined satisfactory level then repeated in spaced intervals and corrective feedback given throughout.

AMERICAN BOARD OF PSYCHIATRY AND NEUROLOGY MAINTENANCE OF CERTIFICATION PROGRAM AS LIFE LONG LEARNING MODEL

Physicians in the United States must demonstrate their engagement in lifelong learning by choosing and participating in CME and in MOC. The MOC program of established by the ABMS requires physicians to base their lifelong learning on self-assessment (SA) and practice-based performance.[24] The Accreditation Council for Continuing Medical Education requires that CME activities that are counted toward a physician's MOC need to be relevant to their practice and contribute to improvements to their strategies, skills, performance, and coordination within health care teams.[25] They also define acceptable outcome measurements for CME activities that focus on changes in physicians' skills or abilities, actual performance on the job, or patient outcomes. The next section describes the history and current status of the ABPN MOC programs in the context of lifelong learning.

BRIEF HISTORY OF AMERICAN RECERTIFICATION AND MAINTENANCE OF CERTIFICATION PROGRAMS

Recertification or time-limited certification discussions are almost as old as discussions of certification. The Advisory Board for Medical Specialties, a precursor to the ABMS, was formed in 1933 and only 7 years later, in 1940, brought up the possibility of time-limited specialty certification.

It was not until 1973 that the successor of the advisory board, the ABMS, formalized the encouragement of member boards to consider measures for assuring continued competence of practicing diplomates through recertification. Early specialties to adopt recertification policies were family practice and internal medicine with family practice being the first to issue time limited certificates beginning in 1976.[26] Psychiatry did not immediately follow suit.

PSYCHIATRY'S ROAD TO RECERTIFICATION

Shortly after the ABMS resolution regarding recertification in 1973, the topic became one of contention in psychiatry with leaders in the field representing diverse opinions from strong support to perhaps even stronger opposition. **Box 3** is a summary timeline of the challenging move of psychiatry and the ABPN toward recertification.[27]

Box 3
Psychiatry's road to recertification

- *1975* A call from a member of the ABPN supports recertification

- *1976* The Group for Advancement of Psychiatry Task Force recommends a focus on getting psychiatrists certified first, and then moving to a voluntary process for periodic certification that might be linked to relicensure.

- *1977* A survey of New York psychiatrists revealing opposition to recertification, although they supported CME requirements.

- *1978* An American Psychiatric Association (APA) is referendum released that recommended, among a number of things, that recertification should be voluntary, offer a number of options for varied practices along with some core material, and methods to include CME, APA SA products and some look at clinical work. It did not endorse ABPN sponsored recertification testing.

- *1979* The ABPN moved to recertify by 1985, but this was movement rejected in 1980 by the ABMS.

- *1981* The ABPN decides to reevaluate and essentially the next several years are filled with many debates about psychiatric recertification with the pro feeling that outside pressures demanded that the field move toward recertification itself, citing the outside pressures from the public and governmental demands and the con basing its rejection on the lack of evidence that certification and/or recertification demonstrated improved competence.

- *1987* The ABPN decides to revisit the issue through the development of a new committee.

- *1989* The ABPN sets the date of October 1, 1994, as the date after which the psychiatry recertification process will be time limited to a 10-year certification and announced that no later than January 1, 2000, a recertification examination would be implemented. Child and adolescent psychiatry time-limited certificates followed 1 year later. Those diplomates with certification before 1994, or 1995 for child and adolescent psychiatry, were given lifetime certification based on legal issues related to possible contract violation, a common policy adopted by other specialties.

Data from Shore J. The Evolving Process of Certification and Recertification. In: Shore JH, Scheiber SC, editors. Certification, Recertification, and Lifetime Learning in Psychiatry. Washington DC: American Psychiatric Press; 1994.

AND THEN, THE LONG EVOLUTION OF MAINTENANCE OF CERTIFICATION, A CONTINUING SAGA

In the early 1990s a number of factors came together to impact the practice of medicine in the United States. Recertification was in full swing. Then Institute of Medicine reports in 2000 and 2001 brought into focus public and political concerns about the state of medical care in the country. These reports highlighted the marked increase in the number of medical errors across the nation, along with the need to make health care more equitable and efficient while improving safety and effectiveness in a more patient centered manner.[27,28] At the same time both the ACGME and the ABMS began to talk about 6 general competencies, including patient care, medical knowledge, practice-based learning and improvement, interpersonal and communication skills, professionalism, and systems-based practice. At that time the ABMS and its member boards begin to change recertification to a process developed with the goal of ensuring continuous competence across specialties that became what we now know as MOC.

The member boards of ABMS decided to move recertification toward a 4-component MOC around 2000, with ABPN implementing its transition to MOC in 2007. The ABPN defined the 4 parts of MOC as follows[26]:

- *Part I: Professional Standing*—a nonsignificantly restricted license to practice medicine.
- *Part II: SA and CME*—a phased in medical knowledge quality improvement cycle requirement that has evolved over time. The requirement initially required completion of an average of 30 specialty specific Category I CME credits per year over the 10-year cycle and 8 hours of SA CMEs awarded for a SA activity. It was theorized that diplomates would identify areas of knowledge weakness that could ultimately guide their selection of CME activities, creating a medical knowledge improvement cycle.
- *Part III: Cognitive expertise*—The recertification examination is meant to be practice relevant with efforts to assess clinical application of knowledge. Diplomates were eligible to take the examination after completing Parts II and IV of the MOC process. As the process has moved from a 10-year process to what ABPN calls continuous certification the test is only one part of continuing certification, making it possible for the diplomate to be certified for an additional 10 years but only with ongoing timely (every 3 years minimal, preferably annually) completion of other MOC requirements along the way.[26]
- *Part IV: Performance in Practice (PIP)*—This component is meant to address quality improvement in the diplomate's individual practice. Diplomates were initially required to complete PIP units that involved both a clinical module and a feedback module. A clinical module requires the diplomate to collect data from 5 cases from a similar category (treatment type, diagnosis, even location of service) from clinical practice, compare their practice with some peer-reviewed best standard of practice, identify areas where practice might be improved, and then check on the implementation success by reviewing another (or the same) 5 cases within a similar category within 1 month to 3 years to see if the practitioner has made improvements. Initially diplomates also were required to complete a feedback module, which could be either patient oriented or peer oriented. The feedback module includes seeking responses from a minimum of 5 peers or 5 patients (or patient families, in the case of child and adolescent psychiatry) to assess practice components that might improve the effectiveness and/or efficiency

of their clinical practices. The diplomate would review the 5 surveys, identify areas for improvement and again reassess through a repeat of the surveys within 1 month to 3 years to ascertain improvement. The ABPN will audit a number of diplomates regarding what they did to achieve these modules, but they will not access any of the specific information, just a description of the process.[26] Professional organizations like the APA and American Academy of Child and Adolescent Psychiatry developed tools with which the diplomates could complete either of these modules, all available for free from either the APA or the American Academy of Child and Adolescent Psychiatry.

This process has evolved throughout subsequent years. Part I, licensure, remains a requirement. In 2014 the ABPN determined that diplomates were falling behind in their MOC and decided that those first in the 10-year certification process would have to do the 300 hours of CME but only 24 hours of ABPN approved SA CME, and 1 PIP module, either clinical or feedback, essentially one 3-year requirement for SA and PIP. These requirements include all those last certified between January 1, 2007, and December 31, 2011. Those certified from January 1, 2012, through December 31, 2015, were entered into a Continuous MOC Program that included 3 cycles of MOC resulting in 3-year requirements of 90 hours of CME, 24 SA CME, and 1 PIP module (either clinical or feedback). The Part III examination is taken in the 10th year. Diplomates with more than 1 certificate may choose to take an examination that continues their certification in both certificates. Only child and adolescent psychiatry diplomates may recertify in child and adolescent psychiatry without recertifying in psychiatry. All the other psychiatry subspecialties must maintain certification in psychiatry and their subspecialty. Continuous MOC continued after 2015 but added a 1-time patient safety activity.[27,28] For specifics regarding approved products to satisfy the full range of MOC activities, consult the ABPN website at https://www.abpn.com/maintain-certification/taking-a-moc-exam/specialty-moc-exams/maintenance-of-certification-in-psychiatry/. Many of these changes in MOC in psychiatry have been the ABPN's response to concerns from the field, continuing in its efforts to balance ABMS requirements with diplomate and psychiatric organizational feedback.

THE NEWEST AMERICAN BOARD OF PSYCHIATRY AND NEUROLOGY MAINTENANCE OF CERTIFICATION INITIATIVE: THE MAINTENANCE OF CERTIFICATION PART III PILOT PROJECT

This year the ABPN launched an ABPN MOC Part II Pilot Project approved by the ABMS as a pilot that if successful will likely be approved by the ABMS and then may become an ongoing alternative in 2022 in lieu of the secure examination.[29] It is scheduled to run for 3 years, that is, from 2019 to 2021. Diplomates who anticipate recertification during these 3 years, 2019, 2020, and 2021, whose ABPN MOC requirements are up-to-date may participate in this program. This pilot project uses timely articles from professional journals in an assessment activity that will offer an additional option for part III of MOC. Initially, the ABPN chose 40 articles from which participants must choose at least 30. Participants must answer correctly at least 4 of 5 multiple choice questions provided with each article that they choose to receive credit for the article. The participant may use the article in an open book fashion to answer the questions. The questions will be written so that they cannot be easily answered by just reading the abstract. In the unlikely situation where a participant fails to answer correctly 4 of the 5 questions for a specific article, the participant can choose an additional article from the 40 provided. In addition to completing part III of MOC, participants will also be awarded 16 hours of SA credit for part II MOC requirements.

NEW INNOVATIONS IN PRACTICE AND THE ROLE FOR ONGOING CONTINUING PROFESSIONAL DEVELOPMENT AND EVALUATION

In keeping with the application of principles of adult learning theory to CPD, our colleagues within psychiatry and other specialties are already engaging in studies of desirability and effectiveness of current CPD practices and innovations in CPD, whether it be specifically for CME credit or, more important, for actual improvement in the quality of care we provide our patients and education we provide our trainees.

A recent cross-specialty national survey of physicians found that physicians want patient-focused and self-directed CPD activities they are already doing on a regular basis to qualify for CME, and that "the highest-rated innovations included a central repository for listing educational opportunities and tracking continuing education credits, an app to award credit for answering patient-focused questions, 5-min and 20-min clinical updates, and an e-mailed 'question of the week.'"[30] The quantity and frequency of initial and reassessment questions and feedback to help maintain knowledge could be based on the RMF technique discussed by Rawson and Dunlofsky as described elsewhere in this article.[22]

With the increasing use of technology across educational settings, including CPD for physicians, Scott and colleagues propose 10 evidence-based principles in the use of technology-enhanced learning in CPD for health care professionals.

> [C]larify purpose and conduct a needs assessment; allocate adequate time and technology; incorporate proven approaches to improve learning; consider the need for a skills component; enable interaction between learners and with others; create different resources for different groups; pilot before implementing; incorporate measures to retain learners; provide opportunities for revision to aid retention; and evaluate learning outcomes, not just satisfaction.[30]

Several specialties rely heavily on simulation-based exercises in residency and fellowship programs and are increasingly doing so in CPD activities. A systematic review of simulation-based CPD activities in acute care specialties found that participants rated these as positive learning experiences, and there was some, although more limited, evidence that they supported improved learning.[31] The study authors recommended ongoing research as to the optimal modality and frequency of these trainings and the translation to actual improved patient care. Although psychiatry is not a procedure-based specialty, simulations, or peer- or expert-evaluated real-life or standardized patient interviews could be similar to a simulation session in allowing participants to practice a skill (eg, deescalation, the physical and psychiatric examination for catatonia or neuroleptic malignant and serotonin syndromes, obtaining information from a patient having difficulty communicating) in real time and obtain feedback on areas for improvement. This would be like the Clinical Skills Verification examination that has now replaced oral boards for psychiatry trainees, and, like the Clinical Skills Verification rather than the oral boards, could occur more often and in the participant's own geographic region, making it more accessible and cost effective, and arguably more relevant.

Within our own field, Murray and colleagues[32] described the use of reflection as a tool in CPD, which follows many of the adult learning principles and desired features of CPD described elsewhere in this article. The authors write, "In keeping with this recommendation to embed activities within the work environment, we suggest a novel application of reflection: structured, peer-facilitated reflection (PFR) as a faculty development strategy to help individuals solve 'real-life' problems while also fostering a community of practice."

The literature seems to support the use of the Kirkpatrick model in assessing the effectiveness of programs[33] (**Table 1**). Most assessments reviewed for this current article seem to stop at the level of reaction and learning, and we continue to need more focus on behavior and results. This discussion hopefully provides a framework for the design of new and assessment of current approaches to help foster lifelong learning for our specialty and beyond.

LIFELONG LEARNING IS A COMPONENT OF PROFESSIONALISM IN PSYCHIATRY

No one questions that the physician must continually work to improve his/her knowledge along with clinical skills to insure the continued provision of quality care for patients. Bard, in his graduation address to the first class of medical students at King's College emphasized that the medical degree was just the beginning of the learning process, while physicians' "whole lives" have to be a work of improvement if they are to achieve their duty to their patients.[34] It is this mantra of maintaining competence across the lifespan that has led to the development of MOC. Although physicians engage in CME, evidence has begun to develop that question whether undirected CME actually facilitates ongoing competence. Typically physicians choose passive types of CME along with topics that appeal to them, not necessarily topics where they have a gap in knowledge.[35] Unguided SA has also been shown to be ineffective.[36] Most studies have demonstrated little, no or an inverse relationship between SAs and external assessments, such as observations or benchmark comparisons. The more concerning finding is that the worse accuracy in SA occurs most frequently among the demonstrably least skilled, yet most confident, physicians.[37] Additionally, studies on pass rates for recertification after the advent of time limited board certification have demonstrated that pass rates decrease the longer the diplomate is from initial certification, suggesting that clinical experience does not ensure being up to date.[38]

Table 1
The Kirkpatrick model

Level 1: Reaction	The degree to which participants find the training favorable, engaging and relevant to their jobs
Level 2: Learning	The degree to which participants acquire the intended knowledge, skills, attitude, confidence and commitment based on their participation in the training
Level 3: Behavior	The degree to which participants apply what they learned during training when they are back on the job
Level 4: Results	The degree to which targeted outcomes occur as a result of the training and the support and accountability package

From Kirkpatrick Partners. The Kirkpatrick Model. Available at: https://www.kirkpatrickpartners.com/Our-Philosophy/The-Kirkpatrick-Model. Accessed May 8 2019; with permission.

SUMMARY

- Model programs in lifelong learning should be designed based on principles of adult learning theory.
- Model programs should tap into the metacognitive processes involved in creating durable knowledge and skills.
- Passive types of CME and unguided SA have been shown to be ineffective.
- The ABPN MOC Pilot Project uses educational techniques that increase the promotion of both durable and efficient learning.
- Lifelong learning within the context of MOC programs will benefit from the innovations emerging from medical education research using technology and assessments strategies.
- All physicians should embrace lifelong learning to enhance improvement in the quality of care we provide our patients and the education we provide our trainees.

REFERENCES

1. The monograph states that "The NHDR and NHQR are the products of collaboration among agencies across the Department of Health and Human Services (HHS). Many individuals guided and contributed to this report." No single author is identified. Available at: https://archive.ahrq.gov/research/findings/nhqrdr/nhqr10/nhqr10.pdf.
2. Institute of Medicine. Crossing the quality Chasm: a new health system for the twenty-first Century. Washington, DC: The National Academy Press; 2001.
3. Institute of Medicine. Improving the quality of healthcare for mental and substance-use conditions. Washington, DC: The National Academy Press; 2006.
4. McGlynn EA, Asch SM, Adams J, et al. The quality of health care delivered to adults in the United States. N Engl J Med 2003;348(26):2635–45.
5. Choudhry NK, Fletcher RH, Soumerai SB. Systematic review: the relationship between clinical experience and quality of health care. Ann Intern Med 2005;142(4): 260–73.
6. Cabana MD, Rand CS, Powe NR, et al. Why don't physicians follow clinical practice guidelines? JAMA 1999;282(15):1458–65.
7. Regnier K, Kopelow M, Lane D, et al. Accreditation for learning and change: quality and improvement as the outcome. J Contin Educ Health Prof 2005;25(3): 174–82.
8. Gilbody S, Whitty P, Grimshaw J, et al. Educational and organizational interventions to improve the management of depression in primary care: a systematic review. JAMA 2003;289:3145–51.
9. Mazmanian P, Davis D. Continuing medical education and the physician as a learner guide to the evidence. JAMA 2002;288(9):1057–60.
10. Davis D, Mazmanian P, Fordis M, et al. Systematic review accuracy of physician self-assessment compared with observed measures of competence. JAMA 2006; 296(9):1094–102.
11. Campbell C, Silver I, Sherbino J, et al. Competency-based continuing professional development. Med Teach 2010;32:657–62.

12. Moore D, How Physicians learn and how to design learning experiences for them An Approach Based on an Interpretive Review of Evidence, From Continuing education in the health professions: improving healthcare through lifelong learning. Proceedings of a conference sponsored by the Josiah Macy, Jr Foundation; 2007 Nov 28-Dec 1; Bermuda [monograph on the Internet]. New York: Josiah Macy, Jr Foundation; 2008. Accessed July 24, 2011.

13. Kolb DA. Experiential learning. Englewood Cliffs (NJ): Prentice Hall; 1984.

14. Armstrong EG, Parsa Parsi R. How Can Physicians' Learning Styles Drive Educational Planning. Acad Med 2005;80(7):680–4.

15. Jennings S. Personal development plans and self-directed learning for healthcare professionals: are they evidence based? Postgrad Med J 2007;83:518–24.

16. Brookfield S. Understanding and facilitating adult learning. Milton Keynes: Open University Press; 1986. p. 96.

17. Eva K. Dangerous personalities [editorial]. Adv Health Sci Educ Theory Pract 2005;10:275–7.

18. Thomson O'Brien MA, Freemantle N, Oxman AD, et al. Continuing education meetings and workshops: effects on professional practice and health care outcomes. Cochrane Database Syst Rev 2001;(2):CD003030.

19. TEAL Center Staff. TEAL center fact Sheet No. 11: adult learning Theories. New York: US Department of Education, Office of Vocational and Adult Education; 2011. Available at: https://lincs.ed.gov/state-resources/federal-initiatives/teal/guide/adultlearning.

20. The Principles of Adult Learning Theory. Available at: https://online.rutgers.edu/blog/principles-of-adult-learning-theory. Accessed April 8, 2018.

21. Hattie J, Donoghue G. Learning strategies: a synthesis and conceptual model. NPJ Sci Learn 2016;1:16013.

22. Rawson K, Dunlosky J. Retrieval-monitoring-feedback (RMF) technique for producing efficient and durable student learning. In: Azevedo R, Aleven V, editors. International handbook of metacognition and learning technologies. Springer Publishing Company; 2013. p. 67–78.

23. Rawson K, Dunlosky J. Optimizing schedules of retrieval practice for durable and efficient learning: how much is enough? J Exp Psychol Gen 2011;140(3):283–302.

24. Miller S. American Board of Medical Specialties and repositioning for excellence in lifelong learning: maintenance of certification. J Contin Educ Health Prof 2005;25:151–6.

25. Holmboe E, Cassel C. Continuing medical education and maintenance of certification: essential links the Permanente. Perm J 2007;11(4):71–5.

26. Certification and Recertification, S. Mouchly Small, in The American Board of Psychiatry and Neurology: The First Fifty Years. In: Hollender M, editor. Deerfield (IL): American Board of Psychaitry and Neurology; 1991

27. Shore J, Schreiber S. The evolving process of certification and recertification. In: SJaS S, editor. Certification, recertification, and lifetime learning in psychiatry. Washington, DC: American Psychiatric Press; 1994. p. 1–18.

28. Aminoff M, Faulkner L, editors. Recertification and maintenance of certification, in the American Board of Psychiatry and Neurology: looking back and moving ahead. Washington, DC: American Psychiatric Publishing; 2012. p. 283–300.

29. American Board of Psychiatry and Neurology, I. MOC Part III Pilot Project. Available at: https://www.abpn.com/maintain-certification/moc-part-iii-pilot-project/. Accessed October 28, 2018.

30. Cook D, Price DW, Wittich CM, et al. Factors influencing physicians' selection of continuous professional development activities: a cross-specialty national survey. J Contin Educ Health Prof 2017;37(3):154–60.
31. Khanduja P, Bould MD, Naik VN, et al. The role of simulation in continuing medical education for acute care physicians: a systematic review. Crit Care Med 2015;43: 186–93.
32. Murray S, Levy M, Lord J, et al. Peer-facilitated reflection: a tool for continuing professional development for faculty. Acad Psychiatry 2013;37(2):125–8.
33. Kirkpatrick Partners. The Kirkpatrick Model. Available at: https://www.kirk patrickpartners.com/Our-Philosophy/The-Kirkpatrick-Model. Accessed September 16, 2018.
34. Bard S. A discourse on the duties of a physician: address to the first graduating class at the medical school established in affiliation with what was then known as King's College. New York: A & J Robertson; 1970. {As cited in Talbott JH, A Biographical History of Medicine, p. 356}.
35. Bowers EA, Girard DE, Wessel K, et al. Barriers to Innovation in Medical Education. J Contin Educ Health Prof 2008;28(3):148–56.
36. Silver I, Campbell C, Marlow B, et al. Self-assessment and continuing professional development: the Canadian perspective. J Contin Educ Health Prof 2008;28(1):25–31.
37. Davis DA, Mazmanian PE, Fordis M, et al. Accuracy of physician self-assessment compared with observed measures of competence: a systematic review. JAMA 2006;296(9):1094–102.
38. Rhodes RS. Maintenance of certification. Am Surg 2007;73:143–7.

Advanced Leadership Training

Pursue an MBA or Other Advanced Degree?

R. Kevin Grigsby, MSW, DSW

KEYWORDS

- Leadership • Management • Organization • Executive • Development
- Graduate degree

KEY POINTS

- Advanced leadership training is available in many forms. Before engaging in formal advanced leadership training, you should engage in a careful and thorough assessment of your motivation for pursuing another credential. You should have a clear understanding of the outcome and impact you desire.
- There are many options, informal and formal, for advanced leadership training. Informal training through mentoring, professional development seminars, and certificate programs will help you to gain leadership knowledge and skills. However, only formal graduate degree programs offer a *bona fide* academic credential. Before enrolling in a graduate degree program, exercise due diligence to be sure this course of action will result in the outcome you desire.
- Selecting your best option should include consideration of cost, financial and personal. Consider the cost of lost opportunities, because pursuit of a graduate degree requires sacrificing your time, effort, and energy. Ask yourself if the potential return on investment (ROI) will be reasonable. Enlisting a neutral third party to assist with calculating the ROI is recommended.
- Check references before enrolling. Speak to persons who have participated or are participating in specific programs before committing to enrollment.

INTRODUCTION

Many articles offer information about basic leadership skills development. This article offers concrete guidance to psychiatrists considering advanced leadership training. Typically, psychiatrists assume leadership roles as they participate in graduate

Disclosure Statement: The author and his family have no direct financial interest in the subject matter or materials discussed in the article or with an organization offering a competing product. The author is solely responsible for the opinions and content and do not represent the views or opinions of the author's employer, the Association of American Medical Colleges.
Member Organizational Development, Association of American Medical Colleges (AAMC), 655 K Street, Northwest, Washington, DC 20001, USA
E-mail address: kgrigsby@aamc.org

Psychiatr Clin N Am 42 (2019) 439–446
https://doi.org/10.1016/j.psc.2019.05.005
0193-953X/19/© 2019 Elsevier Inc. All rights reserved.

medical education and engage in the practice of psychiatry. Although they are expected to demonstrate leadership skills, they may not hold a leadership position and title that connotes formal leadership responsibilities and concomitant accountability. Some of these individuals may demonstrate leadership potential that is largely based on what they have learned "on the job." In turn, they may be selected for a formal leadership position that carries a formal leadership title. However, demonstrating leadership potential is not the same as knowing, doing, and being a leader.[1] In fact, what they have demonstrated may be limited to managerial rather than leadership potential. Leading may look easy, but it is not. In fact, failure is common.[2] Advanced leadership training does not guarantee success. But it is highly likely it improves one's chances of success!

Advancing Your Leadership Skills

This article's target audience is experienced psychiatrists who are considering advanced leadership training. If you are not an experienced psychiatrist, please keep reading because you may find it to be helpful even if you are in an earlier stage of your career. For example, readers who are in the process of considering or applying to medical school have more options than in the past. If you are drawn to medicine and business, you no longer must choose between medical school and the MD degree or business school and the MBA degree. Today, there are 65 joint MD/MBA degrees from which to choose.[3] Typically, these programs require 5 years of full-time study: 3 years of full-time medical curriculum followed by 1 year of full time business school curriculum and a final year of combined study. If you are certain you possess the aptitude, desire, ambition, resources, and stamina to pursue both degrees, it is a viable route to advanced leadership training. If you are uncertain or ambivalent, take heed. It is likely this course of action is not for you.

UNDERSTANDING WHERE YOU ARE AND WHERE YOU WANT TO GO

Before engaging in formal advanced leadership training, you should engage in a careful and thorough assessment of your motivation for pursuing another credential. You should have a clear understanding of the outcome and impact you desire. As mental health professionals, most psychiatrists understand the importance of gaining insight as to our own temperament, preferences, and motivation. The days when every psychiatry resident experienced psychoanalysis as part of training are long gone.

The need for insight, thoughtful reflection, and mindfulness is emphasized during psychiatric training. Knowing "where you are" is critically important as you consider investing in advanced leadership training. You should consider this investment in the same way you consider investing in stock or real estate: it comes at a price, requires time and energy, and carries risk. Risk might be expressed as return on investment (ROI). In the best case, you profit from the investment, or break even. However, you may not reap the rewards for which you hoped. Unlike a stock, you cannot cut your loss by "dumping" and harvesting the residual value. Your personal and financial investment is a sunk cost; it has been incurred and cannot be recovered.

Exploring your motivation to pursue advanced leadership training is critical. In this process, consider drawing on the wisdom of others to learn why you should not pursue advanced leadership training. The Association of MBAs[4] suggests four reasons not to pursue an MBA degree that can be applied to the MHA, MPA, or other graduate degree programs related to leadership in the health enterprise:

1. You are not sure of what else to do.
2. Increasing your salary is your only goal.

3. You think it is the best way to start your entrepreneurial journey.
4. You believe it is necessary to advance your career.

If none of these reasons apply to you, then you should take time to explore formal leadership programs. Invest time to reflect on what is behind your motivation. Pink[5] synthesizes social science research findings about motivation. Three factors drive motivation: (1) autonomy, (2) mastery, and (3) purpose:

- Autonomy is the desire to be self-directed.
- Mastery is the urge to acquire better skills.
- Purpose is the desire for something that has meaning and is important.

It is easy to see how autonomy, mastery, and purpose are behind the drive to complete medical school, residency, and fellowship. Do you have the same level of motivation to complete advanced leadership training? Developing your leadership acumen may result in increased autonomy in terms of developing and operating a practice. You may have great interest in mastering a set of complex business skills, such as stochastic modeling. Completing an advanced degree in business, management, or administration offers an opportunity to master new skills. If you find purpose and meaning in making the world a better place by "improving the health of all," advanced leadership training will help you to enhance your behavioral repertoire.

It is unlikely anyone other than you can determine what is driving your desire to pursue advanced training. Nonetheless, you may find it helpful to have conversations with persons who have completed advanced leadership training because they may help you explore options and become more aware of your own blind-spots. Speak with others about what they hoped to gain from advanced leadership training. Do not be afraid to ask if they gained what they hoped to gain. As best, articulate what you expect to gain given the cost, effort, and attention required. Ask them if your expectations are realistic. Most importantly, generously listen and consider what they say. The admonition to "know before you go" applies here. Do not commit to or engage in advanced leadership training until you have an unambiguous understanding of:

- Your motivation for engaging in advanced leadership training
- What you expect or hope to gain from advanced leadership training
- The sources of support (financial, professional, and personal) you will need to successfully complete the degree

TIMING IS IMPORTANT

You have ascertained you are sufficiently motivated. You are not ambivalent; pursuing advanced leadership training is what you want to do. Now it is time to move on to the next consideration: timing. Do you want to engage immediately? When it is convenient? Soon? Someday? It is important to consider timing early in the process because it may influence the program or structure you choose. Apply due diligence as you develop a plan:

- Is this a "once in a lifetime" opportunity? Does "you snooze, you lose" apply because hesitation may result in losing the opportunity altogether? If this is the case, move swiftly.
- Is the "constellation of events" comprising your life at a point where pursuing advanced training makes sense? Or is this a time where life events may preclude taking on additional activities? If you are expecting the birth or adoption of a child, caring for person with a disability, changing jobs, or relocating, it may be prudent to postpone pursuing advanced training.

- Are you expecting to support a child or children entering college? Tuition and associated expenses represent a significant, long-term financial burden.
- Do you have significant student loan or consumer debt? Most advanced leadership training programs are expensive. Is it wise to accumulate additional debt?

SELECTING THE BEST COURSE OF ACTION FOR YOU

Selecting the best option for advanced leadership training is not simple. Calculating the financial ROI is important. There are also other costs to consider:

- Financial costs you will incur in addition to tuition, such as books and supplies.
- Personal "costs" you will incur in terms of how graduate study will influence your relationships with family, colleagues, and friends.
- Costs of opportunities lost. Will your ROI be worth the benefits you would reap from investing your efforts in other endeavors?
- Travel costs if you are enrolled in distance learning that requires time "in residence."

Can you attain your desired outcome without completing a graduate degree? For example, if your primary interest is in operating a psychiatric practice or developing expertise in reimbursement models, you may not need to commit to completing a degree. There are many on-line or limited duration programs focused on specific aspects of the physician practice enterprise. Typically, these programs result in the award of a formal certificate of completion. They are limited in scope and less intense than graduate degree programs. Financial and personal costs are lower. However, no formal academic credential, such as graduate degree, is awarded on completion. If you are interested in adding an additional set of letters after your medical degree, anything short of pursuing a formal degree is likely to leave you feeling less satisfied.

EXPLORE DEGREE OPTIONS

If you believe your motivation to pursue a degree is sound, the timing is right, and you have the necessary resources, you should explore options. The most common degrees include:

- Master of Business Administration (MBA)
- Master of Health Administration (MHA)
- Master of Public Health (MPH)
- Master of Public Administration (MPA)
- Master of Medical Management (MMM)

Table 1 offers information about the scope of study for each degree and information about the accrediting body and Web site listing accredited programs in each professional discipline.

There are more than 800 Association to Advance Collegiate Schools of Business accredited business schools across the globe and hundreds of MPH, MHA, and MPA programs accredited by AAPHP, Council on the Accreditation of Health Management Accreditation, and Network of Schools of Public Policy, Affairs, and Administration. Highly specialized graduate degrees, such as MMM, targeting physician health care executives are newer options. No matter which degree you choose to pursue, they have many common features including the requirement of a significant investment of time, money, and self. Take time to learn about the advantages and disadvantages offered by each degree. Think about your career aspirations. If you are interested in private sector health enterprises, the MBA may be the best choice. If

	Table 1	
	Graduate degree program accreditation and scope of study	
Discipline/Degree	Accreditation Body and Accredited Programs List	Scope of Study
Master of Business Administration (MBA)	Association to Advance Collegiate Schools of Business International.[6] https://www.aacsb.edu/accreditation/accredited-schools?F_Accreditation=Business	Broad range of topics relevant to any business, such as accounting, finance, management, marketing, economics.
Master of Health Administration (MHA)	Council on the Accreditation of Health Management Accreditation.[7] https://cahme.org/healthcare-management-education-accreditation/students/search-for-an-accredited-program/	Business topics limited in scope to management of health systems and hospitals.
Master of Public Health (MPH)	Association of Accredited Public Health Programs.[8] http://www.aaphps.org/aaphp-member-programs.html	Topics related to management of community health services, such as population health and prevention.
Master of Public Administration (MPA)	Network of Schools of Public Policy, Affairs, and Administration.[9] https://accreditation.naspaa.org/resources/roster-of-accredited-programs/	Management of governmental or quasi-governmental health-related services.
Master of Medical Management (MMM)	Few, accreditation varies across programs	Advanced management skills for physician executives.

your interests relate to inpatient facilities, the MHA may be for you. The MPH degree may be best if you are interested in publicly funded community mental health programs. If you aspire to a leadership position related to mental health services in correctional facilities, the MPA may be a good choice. Experienced physician executives may opt for the MMM degree. Or you may explore the options and decide not to pursue a graduate degree, or at least, not to pursue a graduate degree right now.

IS ACCREDITATION IMPORTANT?

Many graduate programs are accredited by disciplinary societies. Some programs are not accredited. Accreditation is an important consideration because it is the primary means for ensuring and improving the quality of higher education institutions and programs.[10] Not all graduate leadership programs are created equal; reputation matters. Professional colleagues and others will take note of the degree and the institution awarding the degree. Higher status is afforded to accredited programs. Even higher status is afforded to graduate degrees from elite universities. Other programs have found a niche catering to working adults. They are marketed heavily and stress flexibility and convenience. The cost of graduate study is similar whether the program is accredited or not accredited. Over time, some nonaccredited programs become accredited. Until that time, enrolling in a nonaccredited program may have potentially negative consequences in terms of how the degree is perceived by others. Documentation of successful completion comes in the form of a diploma.

Diplomas announce the institution awarding the degree. Others may view it as announcing the quality of your degree. If you are going to invest (heavily) in completing the degree, does it not make sense to protect your investment by attending an accredited program?

CHOOSING A LEARNING FORMAT

Several years ago, completing one of these degrees required full-time matriculation including a period of on campus study. The MBA, MHA, MPH, and MPA continue to be offered in a traditional on-campus format, typically 2 years in duration. Most practicing psychiatrists do not have the freedom, or time, for 2 years of full-time study. Today, potential learners can pursue graduate study without having to enroll as full-time students. Part-time, distance learning, online, and hybrid (online combined with a period of in-residence instruction) MBA, MHA, MPH, and MPA programs are now available. Accelerated executive programs for experienced health care leaders are becoming more common, especially for the MBA. These executive programs are shorter in duration, as are MMM degrees. The learning format may use online instruction, distance learning (videoconference), full-time in-residence learning formats, or some combination. For example, a portion of instruction may be offered using didactic lecture format through live video conference technology. Another portion is offered in self-directed learning online modules, and yet another portion is delivered using live-onsite learning groups comprising individual learners who travel to a single location and spend limited time in-residence.

Choosing a learning format is an important decision. If you have never experienced self-directed online learning, it may be unwise to choose a program that is offered only in that format. Online learning is not for everyone. Take a short course on a topic of interest before committing to a single format. Programs offering instruction on nights and weekends may leave you feeling like you have no time for rest and recovery if you are already employed full-time. Be certain you want to pursue a formal degree because it represents significant financial and personal sacrifice. If you are feeling ambivalent, then it is not the right time for pursuing advance leadership development at this level of intensity.

BEFORE YOU MAKE A FINAL DECISION

Check references before enrolling in any advanced leadership training. Speak to persons who have participated or are participating in specific programs. These individuals offer a better perspective than the program's marketing materials. Try to speak with current participants and program alumni before committing to enrolling in any program. If the program uses a traditional classroom-based approach, ask to sit in on a class or two. Think of yourself as an anthropologist or ethnographer who wants to better understand the nature and culture of the program. It is far better to learn about the program and its nuances before you are paying tuition. You do not want to find yourself immersed in the wrong program. It may be the "right" program for others, but others are not paying your tuition or doing the work required.

CELEBRATING YOUR SUCCESS

Do not wait until you have completed the program to celebrate your success. Create milestones to track your progress, such as completing the first course or completing 1 year of study, and celebrate each time you pass one. If you are working with a learning team or cohort, celebrate together even if you are working in multiple

> **Box 1**
> **Another option: graduate study in the science of leadership**
>
> John Tomkowiak, MD, MOL, is a psychiatrist and Founding Dean of the Elson S. Floyd College of Medicine at Washington State University in Spokane. Before his appointment at Washington State University, he served as dean, acting chair of the Department of Psychiatry and Behavioral Health, and professor of psychiatry at the Chicago Medical School at Rosalind Franklin University of Medicine and Science. He is no stranger to the demands of leadership. John does not hold an MBA or MHA degree. In addition to the MD, he holds a Master of Organizational Leadership (MOL) degree. When I asked John about his motivation to pursue a graduate degree in leadership (MOL) rather than the MBA or MHA he explained he chose the MOL because "It's used every day." It is his belief that all physicians are asked to be leaders. When asked about his early leadership experience, John confessed "I was ignorant." He was surprised by the expectations of others, especially the frequency of situations where he was expected to lead and felt unprepared. A mentor introduced him to the "science of leadership"; he was surprised that there was such a field and it stoked his curiosity. He wanted to gain a better understand the leader's role in creating intellectual curiosity and passion in followers. He also wanted to know more about how to inspire others and how to get them to follow-up on their responsibilities. Likewise, he wants to know "the cold, hard facts" about organizational culture and its consequences. Traditional graduate degrees, such as MBA, MHA, MPH, and MPH, did not have the same promise when it came to what he wanted to learn. When he learned the opportunity to pursue a graduate degree specific to leadership was available, he enrolled in the online MOL program and completed it while he was employed full-time in an executive leadership position.

locations. The relationships you develop with your learning partners will be valuable to you in the future when you need consultation or advice on solving daunting problems.

DISCUSSION

There is a plethora of formal leadership training opportunities that result in the award of a certificate or degree (**Box 1**). Making the decision as to the best option requires careful consideration. Individuals should have a clear understanding as to their motivation for pursuing a certificate or degree. Likewise, they should be able to clearly articulate what they expect to gain given the cost, effort, and attention required. Take the time to speak with persons you trust, especially those persons who may know you better than you know yourself. Their objective observations can offer insight as to whether pursuing an advance degree is the right course of action for you at this time. You may want to seek the opinion of a career or vocational counselor because they are experts in exploring your options and the consequences of your choices. One of Sir William Osler's[11] most well-known aphorisms is: "A physician who treats himself has a fool for a patient." Likewise, physicians who try to function as their own career counselor may be relying on the advice of a fool.

REFERENCES

1. Snook S, Nohria N, Khurana R, editors. The handbook for teaching leadership: knowing, doing, and being. Thousand Oaks (CA): SAGE Publications; 2012.
2. Grigsby RK. Five ways to fail as a new leader in academic medicine. Acad Physician Sci 2010;4–5.
3. MBA Crystal Ball. Why doctors are joining MBA programs 2017. Available at: https://www.mbacrystalball.com/blog/2017/05/31/why-doctors-join-mba/. Accessed November 1, 2018.

4. Association of MBAs (AMBA). Why you should not get an MBA. Available at: https://community.mbaworld.com/looking_to_do_an_mba/f/46/t/341. Accessed November 1, 2018.
5. Pink DH. Drive: the surprising truth about what motivates us. New York: Riverhead Books; 2009.
6. AACSB International. AACSB-accredited universities and business schools. Available at: https://www.aacsb.edu/accreditation/accredited-schools?F_Accreditation= Business. Accessed November 1, 2018.
7. Council on the Accreditation of Health Management Accreditation (CAHME). Search for an accredited program. Available at: https://cahme.org/healthcare-management-education-accreditation/students/search-for-an-accredited-program/. Accessed November 1, 2018.
8. Association of Accredited Public Health Programs (AAPHP). Welcome to the Association of Accredited Public Health Programs. Available at: http://www.aaphps.org/aaphp-member-programs.html. Accessed November 1, 2018.
9. Network of Schools of Public Policy, Affairs, and Administration (NASPAA). Roster of accredited programs. Available at: https://accreditation.naspaa.org/resources/roster-of-accredited-programs/. Accessed November 1, 2018.
10. Council for Higher Education Accreditation (CHEA). Ten ways in which accreditation serves students, society, and the public interest. Available at: https://www.chea.org/sites/default/files/other-content/ten-ways-accreditation-serves.pdf. Accessed November 1, 2018.
11. Osler W, Bean RB, Bean WB. Sir William Osler aphorisms from his bedside teachings and writings. Second printing edition. Springfield (IL): Charles C. Thomas; 1961.

Continuing Professional Development
Reflections on a Lifelong Learning Process

Kenneth P. Drude, PhD[a],*, Marlene Maheu, PhD[b],
Donald M. Hilty, MD, MBA[c,d]

KEYWORDS

- Continuing professional development • Lifelong learning • Self-assessment • CME
- CE

KEY POINTS

- Self-directed continuing professional development (CPD) is a key lifelong responsibility of health practitioners to maintain competencies requiring ongoing performance review and self-assessment.
- The creation and use of an individualized CPD plan with specific goals and identified resources and actions to meet them are critical to meaningful continuing education.
- Several evidence-based methods for self-assessing CPD are identified and discussed.

INTRODUCTION

Continuing professional development (CPD) is a responsibility of practicing health professionals to maintain and enhance their performance and improve health care outcomes. It requires professionals to monitor and reflect on their performance, identify opportunities to improve professional practice gaps, engage in formal and informal learning activities, and make practice changes to reduce or eliminate performance gaps.[1] CPD is a lifelong learning process that begins during graduate and postgraduate education and training and continues after obtaining independent licensure. Although initial professional education and training may be structured, as their careers develop, professionals generally have greater discretion in their learning processes. How practicing professionals approach and respond to ethical and legal CPD

Disclosures: The authors have nothing to disclose.
[a] Private Practice, Wright State University, 642 East Dayton Yellow Springs Road, Fairborn, OH, USA; [b] Telebehavioral Health Institute, Inc., 5173 Waring Road, #124, San Diego, CA 92120, USA; [c] Mental Health, Northern California Veterans Administration Health Care System, 10535 Hospital Way, Mather, CA 95655, USA; [d] Department of Psychiatry & Behavioral Sciences, University of California Davis, Davis, CA, USA
* Corresponding author.
E-mail address: Kenneth.Drude@wright.edu

Psychiatr Clin N Am 42 (2019) 447–461
https://doi.org/10.1016/j.psc.2019.05.002
0193-953X/19/© 2019 Elsevier Inc. All rights reserved.

expectations is generally an individual decision, influenced by personal preferences, practice areas, and possibly explicit licensure and/or certification requirements.

This article reviews the value of CPD and presents some of the ways health professionals can develop, implement, and evaluate their personal CPD during their professional careers. Habits that facilitate CPD, the use of self-refection and self-assessment of practices, developing a personal CPD plan, and obtaining and evaluating the impact of a diversity of learning experiences are presented.

CONTINUING PROFESSIONAL DEVELOPMENT EFFICACY AND BASIS FOR CONTINUING PROFESSIONAL DEVELOPMENT

The benefits of CPD activities have been shown to improve clinical competence and, to a lesser degree, practitioner performance, resulting in improved client/patient health.[2,3] Some forms of continuing education (CE) have greater impact than others on practitioner performance and client/patient health. For instance, Cervero and Gaines[2] (2015), in a study of physician continuing medical education (CME), found that the most effective forms of CE were interactive, used multiple methods, involved multiple exposures, were longer, focused on outcomes, and were considered important by the participants.

In addition to demonstrating initial competency for independent practice, practitioners are increasingly being held to higher standards for relicensure and recertification by changing mandatory CE requirements. These requirements vary considerably across professions and regulatory jurisdictions and often include requirements for specific types of required content and amounts of time. As professional practices evolve, and new standards are adopted, CE requirements are becoming more specific, and, at times, limiting practitioners' choices about how they comply with them. An example of this is the increasing inclusion of telehealth practice in state health professional licensing laws and regulations that may include explicit CE requirements (eg, Georgia Composite Board of Professional Counselors, Social Workers, and Marriage and Family Therapists[4]; Texas Board for Marriage and Family Therapists[5]).

CPD is more than periodically obtaining a minimum number of CE credits. CPD is commonly considered to be a self-directed and planful ongoing process of maintaining and enhancing individual professional competencies as well as the improvement of practice performance. Much of currently mandated CE is didactic, knowledge focused, and as a result may relate little to practitioner performance.[6] In addition to remaining knowledgeable about relevant practices, practitioners must maintain or acquire needed skills and attitudes to retain their ethical and legal requirement for competency maintenance. In a world where educators have struggled for decades to develop pretest and posttest models for assessing change after professional education programs,[7–12] educators have shifted their top-down stance to consider and address the perspective of the learner directly. As a result, and to improve on traditional training models, practitioners are now being urged to learn a variety of clinical skills through a process called lifelong learning (LLL) or the ongoing gaining of knowledge and skills throughout life. LLL is now considered to be crucial to apply knowledge, develop skills, and adjust attitudes for clinical care.[13,14] Practitioners are therefore encouraged to reflect on, learn more about, and solve challenging problems in practice, which requires maintaining a variety of skills (not just knowledge),[15] developing new ones, and fostering a drive for both excellence and learning.

Many fields, disciplines, and professions are also trying to help practitioners adapt to changes in health care (eg, technology), and this trend continues to shape change in graduate education programs. In the future, there will most likely be more online training, simulation, and/or interactive electronic examinations that include technical innovations such as artificial intelligence. In addition, professions are beginning to move from training and follow-up examination steps to a longitudinal series of micro-steps; a culture of weekly to monthly learning rather than a quasiannual or 10-year cycle of recertification based on examinations.[16,17]

Practitioners must recognize and deal with multiple potential barriers for CPD. Even if no negative attitudinal biases exist, other issues may interfere. For instance, time commitments and priorities for other activities may compete for availability to engage in CE activities, especially for extended or multiple CE activities. Other possible factors influencing and obtaining CE include organizational budgeting, personal costs, burnout, not having clear CE goals, work-personal balance, and geographic access.

SELF-CARE: SETTING THE STAGE FOR A CONTINUING PROFESSIONAL DEVELOPMENT PLAN

Nurturing yourself is not selfish – it's essential to your survival and your well-being.
—*Renee Peterson Trudeau*

Although CPD at times may seem like an added burden to an already challenging set of professional demands, it is helpful to keep in mind the positive aspects of CPD activities and motivations for choosing a medical or health care profession. Typically, health care professionals have a strong commitment to help benefit others and a desire to learn, wanting to give back to their profession and to experience having made a meaningful contribution in the life of others.

Professional well-being is not just altruistic care for colleagues but also benefits client/patients, because professionals work best when they care for themselves.[18] The clinical career path can be an exciting and demanding endeavor, which at times can lead to stress and challenge to a professional's well-being. Being attentive to both personal and professional needs ought not be ignored. Regularly engaging in good self-care practices and activities that reduce stress, maintaining a daily routine, reasonable self-expectations, and a balance in personal and professional lives are advised.

DEVELOPING A CONTINUING PROFESSIONAL DEVELOPMENT PLAN

Once health professionals have completed formal education and training they are reliant on self-directed CPD to meet their professional goals and requirements for licensure and certification (**Table 1**). However, this emphasis on self-directed learning can be problematic because of the potential for inaccuracy in identifying learning needs.[19] Namely, when examined, practitioners have shown difficulty in accurately identifying their own deficiencies or weaknesses. More specifically, a review of studies of competency self-assessments found a low relationship between physician self-ratings and external ratings.[20] Davis and colleagues[20] reported, in their review of such studies, that those practitioners with the lowest external competency ratings were consistently the most likely to overestimate their competence. Multiple studies of self-assessments have found the same flaws with self-assessments.[21] The potential bias in self-assessment calls not only for humility but also for alternative sources of input when clinicians assess their own performance. Rather than relying solely on personal judgments, practitioners ought to discipline themselves by not only regularly evaluating their own professional practice and related attitudes but also inviting client/patient and peer review of the practitioner's performance along the same dimensions. To make the process manageable, developing a simple checklist of

Table 1
Components of an individual development/learning plan for professional and personal life

Component	Description	Outcome Measures	Concerns/Bad Signs
Health and Wellness			
Cognitive	Acquiring knowledge via senses	Attention, creativity	Forgetting context or key memories
Social	Meaningful interaction with others	Relationship quality and quantity;	Isolation
Physical	—	Adequate energy	Fatigue
Emotional	Interest, passion and empathy	Coping and presence	Depression
Necessary Self-directed Learning			
Case-based reading	Reread and/or read in depth on challenging issue	Self-efficacy and knowledge improve	Superficial and/or too in-depth passages
Individual journal clubs, webinars	Brief overview of new issue or recap of one	Knowledge and resources	Multitasking
Peer consultation: individual and/ or group	Seeking help, advice, and perspective	Understanding, shared experience	Isolation; rote fixes
CE/CME in-depth course to target area	Depth-based priorities for new interests	Knowledge and skills, tips, and best practices	Cost, time, and failure to apply to cases
Longitudinal series on a topic	Incremental learning with others	Networking, application of information	Inadequate time to prioritize
Self-assessment and Peer Assessment/Reflection			
Our assessment of errors or things we would have done differently	Set aside time to review key decisions and outcomes Diary for logging path	Weigh outcomes over time for perspective and take preventive steps	Errors based on patterns continue and compound problems and bad outcomes

Feedback from client/patients, peers and systems	Ask client/patients periodically Use meetings, conferences for support	Structured time for support, feeling part of, and learning together	Improvement in medical practice (PIP) from American Board of Psychiatry and Neurology (see **Table 2**)
Examination on clinical practice	Objective verification of knowledge and skills	Identify strengths and areas for improvement to plan better	PIP examination from American Board of Psychiatry and Neurology (see **Table 2**)
Data-based feedback	Automated data systems provide input on outcomes and decisions	Perspective on patterns of behavior and positive/negative tendencies	Electronic health record, personal health monitor for client/patient
Mandated Components			
State (eg, pain/palliative care, suicide prevention, ethics)	Obtaining training in specific required topic areas	Improved knowledge and skills about mandated topics	Lack of awareness of need for training
Professional organization based (eg, medical license for psychiatry, ethics)	Stipulation of clinical training in line with clinical competence	Includes a wide range of knowledge, skills, and attitudes	Reports to professional and/or medical board may be frivolous or serious
Certification	Compliance with requirements for certification	Maintenance of certification	Loss of certification

Abbreviation: PIP, practice incentives program.

relevant criteria may be applied to self-review and, similarly, used to solicit client/patient and peer feedback along with a traditional review of individual client/patient outcomes.

CLINICAL MEASURES FOR EVIDENCE-BASED FINDINGS

Practitioners seeking to be rigorous about their professional development may also want to include more objective measures of performance with clients/patients based on competencies/skills, guidelines, practice metrics, and financing mechanisms for those in systems of care. Competencies dovetail with LLL as a part of ongoing practice, and some of the other approaches are easy to build into practice (eg, evidence-based practices in the Veterans' Health Administration).[22]

A rigorous focus on personal competencies may lead to identification of areas of needed additional professional training, the development of health record templates, fidelity measurement, and long-term client/patient outcome metric analysis. Engaging in this process may be easier said than done. Guidelines may be difficult to implement, given that many existing guidelines are intentionally aspirational but lacking in specificity regarding outcome measurement; frequently incomplete, as when considering diverse populations or settings; and contradictory, such as with a client/patient struggling with 3 or more chronic diseases.[23] If it is assumed that the practitioner will conduct standardized assessments to measure targets such as depression severity, psychotic symptoms, or substance use,[24] questions begin to mount:

- How can topics of primary focus for self-review be identified?
  Correct behaviors
  Incorrect behaviors
  Remediation or updates
  Typical complaints from peers?
  Client/patient?
- How much time does it take for the practitioner to complete a self-review?
- How regularly should that optimally be completed?
- How much time does it take for clients/patients/peers to complete any surveys?
- How much time should be budgeted to conduct and review the results of client// patient surveys?
- How can the data be efficiently collected, analyzed, and used?
- Where should the data be kept (cloud, thumb drive at home, office, hard drive)?

BOARD CERTIFICATION AND CONTINUING PROFESSIONAL DEVELOPMENT

Obtaining and maintaining specialty board certification can be a major influence on how health professionals approach CPD. Board certification is among the most important milestones in professionals' lives.[25] The primary purpose of certification and maintenance of certification is to protect the public. It is also a way for specialists to show to their peers and to institutions and organizations that they meet essential standards. The process (an example for psychiatry is outlined in **Table 2**) consolidates years of learning to assess competence as a specialist physician. The initial certification examination entails more knowledge-based than performance-based components, and recertification typically verifies the candidate's up-to-date knowledge of the field. Starting in the early 1990s, the American Board of Psychiatry and Neurology[16] moved to issuing 10-year, time-limited certificates to candidates who had successfully passed part I and part II of the boards and to candidates who had successfully passed subspecialty certification examinations. Individuals also began

Table 2
Examples of current and projected professional organizational/board approach to development in practice (American Board of Psychiatry and Neurology Maintenance of Certification outline)

Component	Current ABPN	Transition from Current Medicine and Psychiatry to 2025 and Beyond	Comment
Part I: Professionalism and Professional Standing	• Active, full, and unrestricted medicine in United States or Canada	Continue	Interstate compacts and innovation across states rare (eg, Veterans' Affairs)
Part II: Lifelong Learning (CME) and SA	• Diplomates choose their own category 1 CME activities. • SA CME activities are selected from the ABPN Approved Products list or diplomates gain credit for up to 2 different types of non-CME SA activity options • SA CME credits contribute to the overall number of CME • Includes a 1-time patient safety activity for those certified in 2016 and after	Technology-structured CME increases Quality improves Integration increases, potentially across systems, and feedback and monitoring may increase Requirements, updates, and other such interventions may increase	There will most likely always be some elective, but selectives will increase because of time, money, and requirements from boards Boards may have more requirements because of showing impact of efforts
Part III: Assessment of Knowledge, Judgment, and Skills	• Take a recertification examination every 10 y	Interactive electronic examinations, over time/longitudinal will be an option to replace formal examinations (eg, 10-y cycles of recertification; American Boards of Psychiatry and Neurology or Anesthesiology)	Microsteps (a culture of weekly to monthly learning) or a quasiannual approach is better for learning and practice (eg, MOC anesthesiology 2018)
Part IV: Improvement in Medical Practice (PIP)	• Diplomates identify and implement areas for improvement based on review of their own patient charts (clinical module) or collect feedback on clinical performance from peers or patients via a questionnaire/survey (feedback module) • Diplomates must select and complete their own PIP activity from the approved products	Annual examinations, or the regular weekly/monthly option, will increase in popularity for a sizable group, but not all will want that option	These better examine practice, offer learning opportunities, and provide timely feedback

Abbreviations: ABPN, American Board of Psychiatry and Neurology; MOC, maintenance of certification; SA, self-assessment.

to participate in a maintenance of certification (MOC) program, which, in combination with the recertification, are vital steps in the process of lifelong learning.

With psychiatry, again, as an example, the American Board of Psychiatry and Neurology (ABPN) requires 4 components in an ongoing fashion. Part I is Professionalism and Professional Standing (eg, unrestricted medical license). Part II is Lifelong Learning (CME; CE for other fields) and Self-Assessment , with free choice of activities except for a 1-time client/patient safety activity for those certified in 2016 and after. Part III is Assessment of Knowledge, Judgment, and Skills via an examination every10 years. Part IV is Improvement in Medical Practice (Practice Incentives Program [PIP]; unique across behavioral health professions but not within medicine), in which diplomates identify and implement areas for improvement based on review of their own client/patient charts (clinical module) or collect feedback on clinical performance from peers or clients/patients via a questionnaire/survey (feedback module). This quality improvement exercise is designed for clinically active physicians to identify and implement areas for improvement within their own practices.

Practitioners' choices for evaluation in this area could dovetail to some degree with clinical interests, individual learning plans, and with boarding requirements, overall. Evaluation selections are done with clients'/patients' input and should focus on a standard measure of a target outcome that is already widely used to capitalize on the evidence base. It should align with regulatory and payor metrics, which shift over time. The measure used should directly shape quality evaluation or clinical decision making. The results should be accessible or be technologically inserted into practitioner notes, if possible, to inform decision making.

Using the ABPN example given earlier, a practitioner's CME could focus on any area, although the PIP portion may fit with the evaluation of care metric (eg, health questionnaire for depression with client/patient and/or peer input). In other areas of medicine, the American College of Cardiology has introduced the Lifelong Learning Portfolio (LLP), largely conducted via technology, and tools such as CardioCompass to search guidelines.[26] The Maintenance of Certification for Anesthesiology uses the MOCA Minute, an interactive learning tool being piloted to replace the cognitive examination. It consists of multiple-choice questions such as those typically on MOC anesthesiology examinations (30 questions per calendar quarter).[17]

CONTINUING PROFESSIONAL DEVELOPMENT PLAN

Individual CPD means having an intentional approach to CE or CME that meets personal professional goals as well as external CE requirements. Knowing one's practice involves the process of ongoing self-assessment previously described that identifies practices that the practitioner seeks to improve, add to their areas of competency, or discontinue.

Deciding on personal goals based on the self-assessment is the next step in developing a CPD plan. Using the SMART approach (ie, writing goals that are specific, measurable, achievable, realistic, and time bound) is a useful time-honored way to describe CPD plan goals that provide clarity and accountability.

The next step in creating a CPD plan is to identify and access resources and learning opportunities to achieve the plan goals (**Table 3** lists examples with some pros and cons for each). This step includes many diverse modalities from formal courses to informal interactions with peers. CE to achieve CPD goals may include a wide range of formal learning opportunities, such as courses, conferences, lectures, workshops, webinars, seminars, and symposia. Documenting or accounting for CE credits

Table 3
Continuing education development activities and resources

Activity/Resources	Pros	Cons
Formal course instruction	Selected topic can be very specific to individual needs, potential to interact with other learners regarding topic Selecting a course requires prioritization and use of resources; purposeful process	Time commitment, registration expense, scheduling, especially if done in person vs online
Webinar attendance	Selected topic can be specific to individual needs, if recorded version is available, easy to schedule	May not offer level of learning relevant to learner, if limited to live presentation may not be easy to schedule
Participation in peer consultation	Provides different practice perspectives (particularly if in a group format) and ideas, can be informal, may be as needed or regular intervals	Time commitment, availability of colleagues for meeting
Conferences and organizational meeting attendance	Interaction/discussion with professional colleagues, content may be timelier than published literature Purposeful, invigorating, and breaks up routine	Cost in travel, registration, lodging, scheduling
Providing supervision	Provides formal instruction and guidance for demonstrating and meeting competency requirements Rewarding and inspiring to work with trainees	Time commitment, availability of supervisor with desirable practice knowledge and skills, possibly expense
Reading professional literature	Remain informed about current research and practices, ease of access, inexpensive with university library access	Time commitment for regular reading, expense if numerous journal subscriptions
Writing professional publications	Motivates to remain current about current research and practices Solidifies and concretizes knowledge	Time commitment, availability of resources
Journal reviewer	Remain informed about current professional research and practices	Time commitment
Making presentations; conducting workshops, seminars; teaching classes	Motivates to remain current about current research and practices Networking is good, particularly in workshops and posters	Time commitment for preparation and presentations, demands remaining up to date regarding current practices

obtained is important for personal tracking as well as for licensure or certification requirements.

Although participation in formal CE or CME modalities is often the major focus of CPD, informal modalities can be important means of achieving individual CPD goals. Informal types of CE may include independent reading of professional literature, peer consultation, peer mentoring, and participating in professional organizations.

Clinicians engaging in informal types of CE may be underappreciated as a valuable way to broaden their professional perspective and learning opportunities. It frequently offers greater flexibility in what it focuses on and in gauging the amount of time and effort it involves. The following are several examples of informal CE for practitioners to consider.

Available and accessible professional information and educational resources have dramatically expanded during the computer age and are used by many health care professionals for CPD. Although younger practitioners may be more receptive to using technology for educational purposes than older practitioners,[27] it remains an important learning mode for all health care practitioners. For example, a recent national survey of board-certified US physicians that recorded what educational technologies they used found that nearly all (97%) used online learning and most (84%) had used simulation-based education for their professional development.[27] Online educational opportunities are not only convenient in terms of time and access but sometimes are available at no cost. For instance, one of the authors of this article recently, during the middle of a work day, attended such a CE-approved webinar sponsored by his liability insurance carrier that provided information about certification of emotional support animals.

A tremendous amount of professional literature is freely available on the Internet. Resources such as PubMed provide practitioners opportunities to find professional publications about specific topics within minutes. Some open access and full text professional publications are readily available at journal sites. Practitioners with academic affiliations can access university libraries at a distance to download articles and request and obtain access to books. Sites such as ResearchGate offer opportunities for sharing information about professional activities and publications.

Practitioners can benefit from engaging in individual or group peer consultation or peer mentoring.[28–30] Regardless of what stage a practitioner's career is at, the use of informal collegial consultation can provide peer feedback, facilitate exchange of alternative perspectives and ideas, and be important in maintaining and improving practice performance. This process can effectively occur in person, or with the use of technology, at a distance. The use of secure teleconferencing for this purpose may be especially useful for practitioners who have few locally available peers.[28]

Actively participating in professional organizations is a major way of remaining informed about current and changing professional practices. Practitioners, clients/patients, professional boards, licensing agencies and (if part of a network or system) many others (eg, payors) in health care shape the definition of quality, its measurement, and its outcomes.[31] Although all efforts theoretically are directed toward good care, sometimes there are competing ideas, preferences, and agendas. Professional organizations play 2 important roles: one in buffering issues that do not align or are in contradiction, and the other in organizing issues by providing updates, translating complex concepts, and providing support (eg, networking, interest groups). In addition to traditional conferences, list serves also offer announcements, job opportunities, and important information about industry standards, codes of ethics, and updates on policies. Usually, institutions (eg, academic centers) and professional organizations usher in changes related to financing, critical incidents, and/or new data that affect how practitioners provide care and leads backward to educational requirements (eg, CE) and at times service changes (eg, Joint Commission[32] 2017).

EVIDENCE-BASED METHODS FOR EVALUATING PROFESSIONAL DEVELOPMENT

With the Internet at every professional's fingertips, almost anyone can find topics of interest to appease their curiosities, but planning, executing, and assessing the success of LLL is an different matter. Organizing training and conducting self-assessment of change for CPD is a challenge for many professionals. The issues are complex. The theory and application of assessment tools for structured, formal assessment of learning at the prelicensure and postlicensure levels for professionals is still in the throes of controversy and approximations to the goal.[6,33]

Despite decades of research focused on evaluating in-person professional development, models for assessing the outcome of training experiences at conferences, conventions, and workshops have failed to lead to widespread usage of program assessment tools.[6] At least as far back as 2002, researchers have documented that more than 90% of professional development programs measure participants' reactions because of issues relating to implementation, cost, and usage rather than a change in knowledge or related behavior.[8,34] Even now, typical evaluations of learners' reactions are collected via so-called smile sheets administered at the end of each program. Such smile sheets typically include aspects of the registration process, the meeting room (too cold, too warm), as well as questions about whether or not the speakers knew their topics, adequately fielded questions, and provided useful handouts. Note that most of the aforementioned factors are not related the learner's change of knowledge, skills, or attitudes about the subject at hand. The formal evaluation of learning, then, is considered a serious challenge that cannot be met by many professional training groups.

In considering self-directed learning and possible self-assessment of behavior change related to learning, learners may want to commit to creating a to-do list related to any learning activity engaged in, rather than simply taking notes on the issues outlined by the speaker. After all, comprehension of concepts is one thing, but engaging in behavior change as the result of that comprehension is quite another. Such a to-do list might be reviewed at regular intervals to assess progress, again, not to measure comprehension of the material in a professional training experience but to assess how well the training activity inspired and motivated or prompted the learner to engage in real-life changes with regard to clients/patients, staff vendors, or other stakeholders.

The current professional training approaches to the assessment of predefined learning objectives for professional training programs are reviewed next and suggestions are presented regarding how professionals can extract self-assessment skills from this self-review.

SELF-ASSESSMENT

Self-assessment of competence is gaining increasing popularity as professionals are seeking new and often technology-based ways to augment their learning. This self-assessment movement is becoming increasingly visible through programs such as the Postlicensure Assessment System (PLAS), developed by the National Board of Medical Examiners and the Federation of State Medical Boards (https://www.fsmb.org/spex-plas/).

The PLAS was developed to assist medical licensing authorities in assessing physicians who have already been licensed. However, it can also be used for self-assessment by professionals seeking a thorough self-review. Assessments available through the PLAS include resources for clinical competence assessment through a network of national assessment programs (https://www.nbme.org/Clinicians/collaborators.html). The assessment tools provided by these programs evaluate the physician's medical knowledge, clinical judgment, and patient management skills. A basic example of such a tool is the Special Purpose Examination administered by computer, which can be found at https://www.nbme.org/clinicians/Spex.html. It is an objective, standardized, cognitive examination of knowledge required for the general practice of medicine. Physicians can be referred to take these assessments by various groups or opt to self-refer to test their clinical knowledge and skills. For details, see https://www.nbme.org/about/index.html.

Other programs have a collaborative relationship with PLAS to offer other performance-based methods of assessment, such as medical record reviews, peer (preceptor) assessment and feedback, patient evaluations, and case-based evaluations of physician care. For details, see https://www.nbme.org/clinicians/collaborators.html.

In an effort spearheaded by researchers in the United Kingdom, researchers examining traditional posttest scoring approaches have been attempting to improve several factors related to such assessment techniques.[34] The most germane to the discussion at hand is that of a self-directed learning activity having an objective tool to determine whether learners might need additional focus after having completed a training experience.

Researchers in the United Kingdom have developed the University College London Scheme for Confidence-Based Assessment to solve a variety of learning assessment challenges.[35] The most relevant aspect of that work to self-assessment is related to the learners' structured focus on the confidence in their selected answers. Theoretic information is provided later to provide a context for why the authors of the current article consider this particular tool to be of direct relevance to self-assessment of learning.

As Gardner-Medwin and Gahan[36] (2003) state:

"To measure knowledge, we must measure a person's degree of belief. Though one could take this as the starting point for a learned debate in epistemology or the application of probability theory, the simple point is perhaps best made by considering some words we use to characterise different states. A student, with different degrees of belief about a statement that is in fact true, may be said to have one of the following:

- Knowledge
- Uncertainty
- Ignorance
- Misconception
- Delusion

The assigned probabilities for the truth of the statement would range from 1 for true knowledge, through 0.5 for acknowledged ignorance to zero for an extreme delusion, i.e. totally confident belief in something that is false. Ignorance (i.e. the lack of any basis for preferring true (T) or false (F)) is far from the worst state to be in." [36(p.147)]

The original reason for developing Gardner-Medwin and Gahan's[36] model was to improve students' study habits. They sought to help students develop an awareness of which answers they lacked confidence in and therefore made lucky guesses for, and helped students identify which areas they could improve with additional study.

Gardner-Medwin and Gahan[36] further explained:

"Reflection strengthens links between different strands of knowledge, both before and after feedback - checking an answer or viewing it from different perspectives before placing what is essentially a bet under the confidence-based marking scheme. It strengthens the ability to justify an answer, one of the essential elements in an Aristotelian definition of knowledge (as justified true belief) that is often missing in students who prefer rote-learning to understanding." [36(p. 148)]

Students reportedly have embraced the model, explaining that it helps them identify areas where they have inadequate knowledge. It helps them reflect on their answers and consider additional focus for self-development. This posttest assessment technique has found success in eLearning, as shown by its incorporation into digitized content management software such as the open source Moodle software, commonly used by colleges and universities internationally. The model can be used for any type of answer that can be marked as definitely either right or wrong using answers that are true/false, multiple choice, extended matching sets, text, numbers, or quantities.

Each time an answer is entered, it is followed with a request for the learners to rate their levels of confidence in their selected responses. Readers interested in examining this approach are invited by Gardner-Medwin and Gahan[36] to sample the model in this browser-based version of their software: http://www.ucl.ac.uk/lapt/laptlite/

Practitioners embarking on a path of lifelong learning may want to consider their own confidence levels in the professional development they embrace, and check themselves on their processes when completing posttest items. If they are fortunate enough to have found learning programs that offer confidence-based assessment, they can benefit from noting their own scores that are reflective of guessing at answers to questions that are particularly germane to their own goals for professional development.

If they have to keep track of such guesswork without the assistance of a posttest that is preconfigured to help them conduct this type of self-assessment, they may wish to keep track of such confidence levels in a separate document, so as to be reminded to remediate their self-identified deficiencies before embarking on professional service delivery, in which clarity may be essential to the well-being of a client/patient relying on the practitioner's professionalism.

SUMMARY

CPD is a lifelong learning process that requires health professionals to consider their basic personal welfare needs, professional goals, and self-assessment of current practices, creating a plan for maintaining and/or developing practice competencies and compliance with ethical and regulatory requirements. Given the difficulties in performing unbiased self-assessments, it is important that practitioners obtain information, data, and feedback from other sources, such as client/patient and peers, and any relevant and available clinical or outcome data. An individualized CPD plan to organize this process can provide structure and a format for ongoing reassessment and identifying areas for needed change.

CPD plans need to be regularly reviewed and updated to be responsive to changes in personal, professional, and patient needs and changes in best practices. Finding and accessing formal and informal CE opportunities and resources to meet identified CPD goals is an ongoing process that goes beyond obligations to meet mandatory CE credits for licensure or certification. It requires personal review and reflection by practitioners about their current practices and consideration about what knowledge, skills, and attitudes need to be learned to optimize professional performance. Several evidence-based forms of self-assessment are identified that offer ways for practitioners to evaluate their CPD efforts.

REFERENCES

1. Campbell C, Silver I, Sherbino J, et al. Competency-based continuing professional development. Med Teach 2010;32(8):657–62.
2. Cervero RM, Gaines JK. The impact of CME on physician performance and patient health outcomes: an updated synthesis of systematic reviews. J Contin Educ Health Prof 2015;35(2):131–8.
3. Stevenson R, Moore DE. Ascent to the summit of the CME pyramid. JAMA 2018; 319(6):543–4.
4. Georgia Administrative Code Chapter 135-11 Rule 135-11-01, Telemental Health, 2015. http://rules.sos.state.ga.us/gac/. Accessed November 9, 2018.
5. Texas Administrative Code Title 22, Part 35, Chapter 801, Subchapter C, Rule 801.58 (d) §, Technology-Assisted Services, March 26, 2017. https://texreg.sos.state.tx.us/public/readtac$ext.TacPage?sl=R&app=9&p_dir=&p_rloc=&p_tloc=&p_ploc=&pg=1&p_tac=&ti=22&pt=35&ch=801&rl=58. Accessed November 5, 2018.
6. Kirkpatrick DL, Kirkpatrick JD. Evaluation training programs: the four levels. 3rd edition. Oakland, CA: Berrett-Koehler Publishers, Inc; 2006.
7. Gall MD, Gall JP, Borg WR. Educational research: an introduction. 7th edition. Boston: Allyn & Bacon; 2003.
8. Lynch KB. When you don't know what you don't know: evaluating workshops and training sessions using the retrospective pretest methods. Paper presented at the meeting of the American Evaluation Association Annual Conference. Arlington, VA, 2002, November 6–9.
9. Hill LG, Betz DL. Revisiting the retrospective pretest. Am J Eval 2005;26(4): 501–17.
10. Lamb T. The retrospective pretest: an imperfect but useful tool. The Evaluation Exchange 2005;XI(2), p. 18. Available at: https://archive.globalfrp.org/var/hfrp/storage/original/application/d6517d4c8da2c9f1fb3dffe3e8b68ce4.pdf.
11. Martineau J, Hannum K. Evaluating the impact of leadership development: a professional guide. Greensboro (NC): Center for Creative Leadership; 2004.
12. Nimon K, Allen J. A review of the retrospective pretest: implications for performance improvement evaluation and research. Workforce Education Forum 2007;44(1):36–55.
13. Mohr NM, Moreno-Walton L, Mills AM, et al. Generational influences in academic emergency medicine: teaching and learning, mentoring, and technology (part I). Acad Emerg Med 2011;18(2):190–9.
14. Callan JE, Maheu MM, Bucky SF. Crisis in the behavioral health classroom: enhancing knowledge, skills, and attitudes in telehealth training. In: Maheu MM, Drude KP, Wright SD, editors. Career paths in telemental health. Cham (Switzerland): Springer; 2017. p. 63–80.
15. Iobst WF, Sherbino J, Cate OT, et al. Competency-based medical education in postgraduate medical education. Med Teach 2010;32(8):651–6.
16. Maintenance of certification. American Board of Psychiatry & Neurology. Available at: https://www.abpn.com/maintain-certification/. Accessed February 24, 2018.
17. MOCA Minute®. American Board of Anesthesiology. Available at: http://www.theaba.org/MOCA/MOCA-Minute. Accessed February 10, 2018.

18. Haskins J, Carson JG, Chang CH, et al. The suicide prevention, depression awareness, and clinical engagement program for faculty and residents at the University of California, Davis Health System. Acad Psychiatry 2016;40(1):23–9.
19. Duffy FD, Holmboe ES. Self-assessment in lifelong learning and improving performance in practice: physician know thyself. JAMA 2006;296(9):1137–9.
20. Davis DA, Mazmanian PE, Fordis M, et al. Accuracy of physician self-assessment compared with observed measures of competence: a systematic review. JAMA 2006;296(9):1094–102.
21. Dunning D, Heath C, Suls JM. Flawed self-assessment: implications for health, education, and the workplace. Psychol Sci Public Interest 2004;5(3):69–106.
22. U.S. Department of Veterans Affairs. Spotlight on evidence-based practice (EBP) 2018. Accessed on https://www.hsrd.research.va.gov/news/feature/ebp.cfm. Accessed September 25, 2018.
23. Garber AM. Evidence-based guidelines as a foundation for performance incentives. Health Aff (Millwood) 2005;24(1):174–9.
24. Hilty DM, Turvey C, Hwang T. Lifelong learning for clinical practice: how to leverage technology for telebehavioral health care and digital continuing medical education. Curr Psychiatry Rep 2018;20(3):15.
25. Roberts LW, Hilty DM. Approaching certification and maintenance of certification. In: Roberts LW, Hilty DM, editors. Handbook of career development in academic psychiatry and behavioral sciences. 2nd edition. Washington, DC: American Psychiatric Publishing Incorporated; 2017. p. 325–34.
26. Zoghbi WA, Beliveau ME. President's page: lifelong learning in the digital age. J Am Coll Cardiol 2012;60(10):944–6.
27. Cook D, Blachman M, Price D, et al. Educational technologies for physician continuous professional development: a national survey. Acad Med 2018;93(1):104–12.
28. Paulson LR, Casile WJ, Jones D. Tech it out: implementing an online peer consultation network for rural mental health professionals. Rural Ment Health 2015;39(3–4):125–36.
29. Carney J, Jefferson J. Consultation for mental health counselors: opportunities and guidelines for private practice. J Ment Health Couns 2014;36(4):302–14.
30. Waltman SH, Frankel SA, Williston MA. Improving clinician self-awareness and increasing accurate representation of clinical competencies. Pract Innov (Wash D C) 2016;1(3):178–88.
31. Shi L, Singh DA. Delivering health care in America: a systems approach. 6th edition. Burlington (MA): Jones and Bartlett Learning; 2015.
32. The Joint Commission. Measurement-based care in behavioral health 2017. https://www.jointcommission.org/assets/1/6/bhc_Joint_Commission_measures_webinar_041117.pdf. Accessed September 24, 2018.
33. Chang R, Little TD. Innovations for evaluation research: multiform protocols, visual analog scaling, and the retrospective pretest–posttest design. Eval Health Prof 2018;41(2):246–69.
34. Sugrue B, Kyung Kim K. State of the industry report. Alexandria (VA): ASTD Press; 2005.
35. Bryan C, Clegg K. Innovation assessment in higher education. New York: Routledge; 2006.
36. Gardner-Medwin A, Gahan M. Formative and summative confidence-based assessment. Proceedings of the 7th Computer-Aided Assessment Conference. Loughborough, 2003, July, 147–155.

Embracing Diversity and Inclusion in Psychiatry Leadership

Kari A. Simonsen, MD[a],*, Ruth S. Shim, MD, MPH[b]

KEYWORDS

- Inclusivity • Diversity • Psychiatry • Leadership • Equity • Pipeline • Culture
- Humility

KEY POINTS

- Embracing diversity and inclusion are essential to the practice of high-quality psychiatry, and these tenets also apply to developing and sustaining a diverse and inclusive field of academic psychiatry leaders.
- Pipeline programs for students and medical trainees can provide supportive communities that enhance student success and increase physician diversity.
- Individual leadership development programs provide ongoing faculty development to encourage leadership readiness and effectiveness.
- Organizational policies and development programs are needed to enhance inclusivity in academic medicine.

INTRODUCTION: THE IMPORTANCE OF CULTURE, DIVERSITY, AND INCLUSION IN PSYCHIATRY

There is a growing recognition that culture, diversity, and inclusion are essential to the practice of high-quality clinical care in medicine and, more specifically, in psychiatry. The landmark *Supplement to Mental Health: A Report of the Surgeon General*, entitled *Mental Health: Culture, Race, and Ethnicity*, was one of the first federal reports to provide clear documentation of mental health disparities and how they can be viewed through the lens of culture.[1] Despite this landmark publication drawing attention to the importance of diversity and inclusion, cultural psychiatry has often been viewed as a niche topic within psychiatry,[2] rather than an important and relevant skill for all psychiatric clinicians. In recent years, mental health equity has become an increasing

Disclosure Statement: No relevant disclosures.
[a] Pediatric Infectious Diseases, University of Nebraska Medical Center, 982162 Nebraska Medical Center, Omaha, NE 68198-2162, USA; [b] Department of Psychiatry and Behavioral Sciences, University of California-Davis, 2230 Stockton Boulevard, Sacramento, CA 95817, USA
* Corresponding author.
E-mail address: kasimonsen@unmc.edu

Psychiatr Clin N Am 42 (2019) 463–471
https://doi.org/10.1016/j.psc.2019.05.006
0193-953X/19/© 2019 Elsevier Inc. All rights reserved.

psych.theclinics.com

topic of interest, as reflected by a significant increase in publications about the issue and a significant increase in presentations at national conferences on the importance of mental health equity, diversity, and inclusion.[3] With this renewed attention, it is important to consider why an emphasis on diversity and inclusion in psychiatry, particularly in psychiatric leadership, is critical to improving outcomes for people with mental illnesses and substance use disorders.

Health disparities are defined differences in health care quality that are not due to access-related factors or clinical needs.[4] Health inequities, on the other hand, are driven by societal organization, "giving rise to forms of social position and hierarchy, whereby populations are organized according to income, education, occupation, gender, race/ethnicity, and other factors."[5] Implicit in this definition is the moral imperative that health inequities (and mental health inequities) are unjust and preventable. Findings from the *Mental Health: Culture, Race, and Ethnicity in 2002* show that mental health disparities follow a somewhat different pattern than health disparities related to certain physical illnesses. Compared with white populations, racial/ethnic minorities have poorer access to care, poorer quality of care, and greater disability associated with mental illnesses.[1] Precisely because mental health disparities and, more accurately, inequities persist, cultural competence as a framework with which to consider health disparities has been promoted. A foundational understanding of culture also helps providers understand that patients bring many aspects of their identity into clinical encounters.

Over the past half-century, the theories describing culture in psychiatry have evolved and changed, and seeking to understand these frameworks provides additional context for contemplating the role of culture in psychiatry today. *Cultural competence* has been an extremely important contribution to medicine and has led to heightened awareness of the importance of culture in medicine. Furthermore, cultural competence has helped to improve health outcomes for patients and enhance the quality of care that providers administer.[6] However, cultural competence itself cannot consistently account for intersectionality or complexity associated with culture.[7] As a result, mandatory trainings in cultural competence often lead to reductionist stereotypes about certain racial/ethnic cultural groups (eg, Latino populations have big, close knit families and African Americans are highly religious). In response to these limitations in cultural competence, Melanie Tervalon and Jann Murray-García moved beyond cultural competence to coin the term "cultural humility," which considers principles such as committing to lifelong learning, recognizing power imbalances in medical encounters, and engaging with communities.[8] When reflecting on the importance of diversity and inclusion in psychiatric leadership, the role of power imbalances becomes critical to conceptualizing culture in psychiatry. The current power balance in psychiatric leadership is not representative of the population of patients served by mental health services in the United States. For example, of the 147 presidents of the American Psychiatric Association, only one has been African American (the current president in 2018–2019, Altha Stewart, MD) and only 8% have been women.[9,10]

One tangible metric of the long-standing inequities in academic medicine is faculty salaries, with male primary care physicians earning nearly 18% more than female primary care physicians and male specialist physicians earning 36% more than female specialist physicians.[11] These inequities persist even when adjusting for full-time equivalents, specialty, and work distribution (clinical, research, teaching, administration) and persist despite knowledge of this issue for decades.[12]

When leadership lacks diversity, the policies and norms that are set by leaders may be limited in scope and may skew toward devaluing the importance of diversity and inclusion.[13] This has led to shameful diagnostic and clinical errors in psychiatry, including diagnoses such as drapetomania,[14] pathologizing homosexuality,[15] and, more recently, overdiagnosing schizophrenia in African Americans[16] and psychopathologizing transgender individuals.[17] Representation in leadership in psychiatry is critical to making sure well-meaning providers do not inadvertently set policies or define societal norms based on structural discrimination or without considering important cultural contextual factors.

As cultural humility has evolved, the term "structural competence" has also gained prominence. Structural competence incorporates the social determinants of health into a framework to provide perspective on health inequities.[18] When comparing cultural and structural competence, it is important to consider context, as the level of intervention for cultural competence is usually individual patients and providers, whereas the level of intervention for structural competence is often institutions and policies.

Taken together, these 3 separate frameworks (cultural competence, cultural humility, and structural competence) allow providers to take a more nuanced approach to considering culture in health and psychiatric care. Psychiatrists have moved toward structural competence through regulatory guidance for their trainees, such as the Liaison Committee on Medical Education (LCME) standards around learning about culture, diversity, and inclusion as a requirement of medical school education, and new core standards requiring residency training programs to address diversity and inclusion by the Accreditation Council for Graduate Medical Education (ACGME).[19] However, without leadership that values diversity, inclusion, and representation and then reflects this representation actively within senior leadership in psychiatric organizations, little true and effective progress will be made.

FIRST STEPS: THE PIPELINE FOR PHYSICIAN TRAINING

The Association of American Medical Colleges' (AAMC) most recent annual data on medical school applicants and matriculants demonstrate an acceptance rate of 41.1% overall in 2015. However, acceptance rates differ among select racial/ethnic subgroups, with Asian, Latino/Hispanic, and White applicants having similar acceptance rates (42%, 42%, 44%, respectively) while African American or Black applicants were accepted at a lower rate of 34%.[20] These data show even greater inequities when considering the total percentages of medical school graduates by race and ethnicity. Numbers remained relatively stable from 2011 to 2015 for Asians (19.8%) and Whites (58.8%), together representing almost three-fourth of medical school graduates, whereas only 5% of 2015 medical school graduates were of Latino or Hispanic ethnicity, and 6% were Black or African American.

An important first step to enhance the diversity of academic organizations is through pipeline programs for underrepresented students.[21] Despite knowledge and understanding that increasing provider diversity is a critical element in addressing disparities in health care access and delivery, and health outcomes for minority populations, we continue to contend with a lack of progress in attracting Underrepresented in Medicine (URM) students to academic careers.[22] Gaps in access for URM students earlier in their educational trajectory to explore health careers have been identified as a contributing factor, as are equitable access to resources for successful postsecondary and medical school applications.[23]

A lack of supportive role models and mentors (themselves from URM backgrounds), limited networking opportunities, and institutional and structural discrimination can compound barriers for URM students toward careers in academic medicine.[24]

Unfortunately, this underrepresentation persists when considering medical school faculty, where gender inequities are prominent, with women comprising just 39% of full-time academic faculty (despite accounting for nearly 50% of medical school graduates). Furthermore, only 4% of full-time female academic faculty identify as Black or African American, Hispanic or Latino, Native American or Alaska Native, and Native Hawaiian or Pacific Islander.[25]

Pipeline programs should begin early in the educational continuum for greatest impact in reaching target students within the community to drive engagement, understanding, and visibility of careers in medicine. Programs that begin at the high school level such as the University of Nebraska Medical Center High School Alliance program cultivate interest in health careers with promising high school students, with a mission to increase diversity of the students in the health professions. Results to date indicate greater than 70% of students who complete the program choose a health science undergraduate major.[26]

Undergraduate and post-baccalaureate programs also support URM students in entering health professions careers. For example, Southern Illinois University's Medical and Dental Education Program supports students with both academic and professional development activities, immersive learning environments, and mentoring from physicians and scientists who can serve as future mentors and sponsors. These activities can directly affect barriers as stated by undergraduate students with an interest in pursuing health professions careers.[23]

Pipeline support must continue throughout graduate medical education as well, if we are to be successful in expanding the representation of URM physicians within psychiatry and other medical specialties. The updated ACGME requirements for resident education incorporates specific knowledge and skills in leadership development, team-based medical care, system-based practices, and an understanding of and sensitivity in supporting best practices in the care of diverse patients and populations.[27] Within psychiatry, the Residency Review Committee program milestones provide oversight and evaluation of programs on resident physician educational outcomes including demonstration of knowledge, sensitivity, and commitment to serving diverse patients and populations (defined herein as unique aspects including gender, age, socioeconomic status, race, religion, culture, disability, and sexual orientation) and understanding of and dedication to reducing health care disparities.[28]

DEVELOPING AND SUPPORTING A DIVERSE AND INCLUSIVE FACULTY

Considering the significant underrepresentation at the academic faculty level, additional efforts are required to recruit, retain, and advance URM physicians in academia. One approach many institutions have used as a means to increase visibility in addressing diversity and inclusion activities on campus is through executive leadership with the creation of a position of Chief Diversity Officer (CDO). The rationale for this approach is one that suggests that a senior level leader would have positional authority to increase the diversity of the faculty through power and influence. Unfortunately, emerging evidence does not verify this hypothesis. West and colleagues reviewed data on faculty diversity from 462 US research institutions (Carnegie R1, R2, or M1 designated and >4000 undergraduates) that created a dedicated CDO position. In their analyses, they were unable to identify a statistically significant increase in faculty diversity defined as new faculty hires on a tenure or nontenure track, hiring of tenured faculty, nor for hiring university administrators during the periods before and after creation of a CDO position.[29] Despite the absence of return on investment as defined by greater faculty diversity, over the study period (2001–2016) the momentum continued in developing CDO positions with two-thirds of the potential institutions within the sample creating a CDO position by 2016. Because of the significance of representation and visibility, the benefits of faculty who are URM occupying high-level institutional leadership positions may be difficult to quantify but undoubtedly has an impact on URM medical students, residents, and junior faculty to see leaders who reflect their own racial/ethnic and/or gender backgrounds.

Another broadly applicable intervention to support and promote diversity, equity, and inclusion consists of training programs to increase understanding of the role of implicit bias in perpetuating racial/ethnic and gender inequities. Specific implicit bias training interventions include training for search committee members, bystander training within the clinical and learning environments, and targeted training on bias and the impact of microaggressions for academic senior leadership. Although many academic settings are beginning to implement these trainings at their institutions, they are by no means universal. Significant positive outcomes in educating providers about the dangers of implicit bias in clinical settings have been shown,[30,31] but these findings have not been extensively explored in relation to interventions for hiring and retaining URM faculty or in addressing social exclusion in academic climates. In addition, much like past attempts to train providers in the importance of cultural competence, when bias trainings are conducted by individuals without proper understanding of the complexity of these topics (including issues related to structural racism, privilege, and fragility), efforts to teach people to recognize and mitigate their biases can backfire.[32] In many ways, these controversial findings help to confirm the importance of having enough diverse members of faculty and students within an institution so that harmful or dangerous methods of teaching can be properly identified and addressed before major damage can be done. Furthermore, as experts in human behavior, psychiatrists should lead medicine in efforts to understand the role of implicit bias, its origins, and ways to address and confront bias in order to increase diversity and improve inequitable outcomes in health.

Individual leadership development programs for faculty at all levels also exist to expand the pool of effective leaders within academic medicine. The AAMC provides numerous leadership development courses, including through their Group on Diversity and Inclusion and the Group on Women in Medicine and Science that target URM academic faculty who have the support of their institutions to develop their leadership potential.[33] The AAMC leadership development content areas range from programs for assistant professors to dedicated programs for deans and chief medical officers. One relevant example is the AAMC Healthcare Executive Diversity and Inclusion Certificate Program, which is designed to enhance diversity education competencies of organizational leaders linked directly to challenges facing participant institutions.[34] Another example of a faculty leadership development program specific to women in medicine and science is the Executive Leadership in Academic Medicine (ELAM) program, housed at Drexel University. During more than 20 years the program has existed, more than 1000 women have been trained for senior leadership roles in academic medical centers. Among ELAM graduates, 15% identify as racial and/or ethnic minorities.[35]

WAYS FORWARD: IMPLICATIONS FOR PSYCHIATRIC LEADERSHIP AND THE FUTURE OF PSYCHIATRY

Although there are many viable paths to increase the diversity of psychiatric leadership in academic medicine (and the field as a whole), many challenges exist. Structural discrimination, bias, and stereotypes perpetuate the image of one-dimensional psychiatrist leaders (ie, Sigmund Freud). For significant progress to be made, leaders in psychiatry must begin to better resemble an increasingly diverse field of psychiatry residents who serve a more diverse community of patients.

Within academic psychiatry departments, it is critical that leadership emphasize the importance of diversity through creation and support of committees and policies to advance diversity, equity, and inclusion. The University of California Davis Diversity Advisory Committee is just one example of ways to prioritize diversity initiatives in a Department of Psychiatry,[36] but many departments have successfully implemented unique methods for emphasizing and highlighting the importance of diversity and equity within their programs. Diversity initiatives can also incorporate robust didactic and clinical experiences that explore the structural origins of mental health inequities in outcomes and in leadership. In addition, clearly understanding of the role of implicit bias and privilege will allow departments to improve processes for selecting and recruiting diverse residents and faculty to their programs. Sustainable processes will also incorporate supportive institutional policy changes, including such considerations as salary equity, leave policies, and promotion and tenure guidance, that consistently support individual faculty and build an affirming and welcoming climate.

Sponsorship of women and URM faculty is another essential component to bringing forward more diverse and inclusive leadership in Psychiatry. Specific tactics for sponsors, whether institutions or individuals, should include insisting on nomination of a diverse pool of candidates for awards, when extending offers for speaking opportunities, particularly for high-level, keynote or named lectureships, and for opportunities to be interviewed for perspective and media exposure. Amy S. Gottleib, MD and Elizabeth L. Travis, PhD stated in *Academic Medicine*, "Formal Sponsorship programs

---

Box 1
Ten recommended actions for institutions and individuals to support inclusivity, diversity, and equity in psychiatry

Individual Actions

1. Mentor students and trainees who increase the diversity of programs and support local pipeline efforts.

2. Participate in, support, and lead programs to raise awareness and address implicit biases.

3. Understand the evidence describing disparities faced by women and URM faculty in the medical workforce, use evidence to enact change.

4. Sponsor women and URM faculty for leadership positions, awards, and speaking opportunities.

5. Actively mitigate microaggressions in the workplace that undermine physician productivity, faculty retention, and effective patient care.

Institutional Actions

6. Harness regulatory opportunities and metrics (such as from LCME and ACGME) to actively advance inclusivity at all levels of the institution.

7. Mandate inclusion of diverse membership on institutional committees including major search committees.

8. Use administrative leadership positions, such as Chief Diversity Officer, to convene people across all levels of the organization to advance inclusivity.

9. Institute policies that demand diverse finalists for leadership positions and awards.

10. Institute policies that ensure salary equity.

that match women with senior leaders facilitate access to beneficial relationships and institutionalize the value of equal opportunity."[37]

Ensuring an organizational culture in academic settings that not only follows regulatory guidance from LCME and/or ACGME surrounding developing cultural awareness and humility in our trainees but also extends that cultural humility among the faculty and elevates diverse educational leadership will benefit all our students, the future workforce, and the health of our communities. Engaging psychiatry leaders and institutional administrators, including CDOs, in building inclusive organizational cultures illuminates pathways toward achieving health equity in our patients and communities; specific ways forward are highlighted in **Box 1**.

There are significant implications from a lack of diversity to the future field of psychiatry and to psychiatric leadership. Demographics in medical school education and psychiatry training programs are shifting to reflect greater diversity over time. However, this shift has not led to greater diversity in psychiatric leadership. Without acknowledgment and consideration of the growing diversity, inclusion, and equity in psychiatry, the gulf between mature providers and those medical students, residents, and early career psychiatrists who value these issues continues to grow and may lead to a disconnection in values in psychiatry. There is a danger that a field that resists acknowledging this shift in focus may be at risk for stagnating and losing relevance in modern medicine.

REFERENCES

1. US Department of Health and Human Services. (2001). Mental Health: Culture, Race, and Ethnicity—A Supplement to Mental Health: A Report of the Surgeon General. Rockville, MD: U.S. Department of Health and Human Services, Substance Abuse and Mental Health Services Administration, Center for Mental Health Services. Available at: https://www.ncbi.nlm.nih.gov/books/NBK44243/pdf/Bookshelf_NBK44243.pdf.

2. Lewis-Fernandez R, Kleinman A. Cultural psychiatry: theoretical, clinical, and research issues. Psychiatr Clin 1995;18(3):433–48.

3. Shim RS, Kho CE, Murray-García J. Inequities in mental health and mental health care: a review and future directions. Psychiatr Ann 2018;48(3):138–42.

4. Smedley BD, Stith AY, Nelson AR, editors. Unequal Treatment: Confronting Racial and Ethnic Disparities in Health Care. Institute of Medicine (US) Committee on Understanding and Eliminating Racial and Ethnic Disparities in Health Care. Washington (DC): National Academies Press (US); 2003. Available at: https://www.ncbi.nlm.nih.gov/pubmed/25032386.

5. World Health Organization. Social determinants of health 2017. Available at: http://www.who.int/social_determinants/en/. Accessed April 10, 2019.

6. Truong M, Paradies Y, Priest N. Interventions to improve cultural competency in healthcare: a systematic review of reviews. BMC Health Serv Res 2014;14(1):99.

7. Kumagai AK, Lypson ML. Beyond cultural competence: critical consciousness, social justice, and multicultural education. Acad Med 2009;84(6):782–7.

8. Tervalon M, Murray-Garcia J. Cultural humility versus cultural competence: a critical distinction in defining physician training outcomes in multicultural education. J Health Care Poor Underserved 1998;9(2):117–25.

9. Hirshbein LD. History, memory, and profession: a view of American psychiatry through APA presidential addresses, 1883–2003. Am J Psychiatry 2004; 161(10):1755–63.

10. Presidents of the American Psychiatric Association. Available at: https://en.wikipedia.org/wiki/Presidents_of_the_American_Psychiatric_Association. Accessed April 10, 2019.

11. Medscape. Compensation in medicine 2018. Available at: https://www.medscape.com/slideshow/2018-compensation-overview-6009667#14. Accessed April 10, 2019.

12. Freund KM, Raj A, Kaplan SE, et al. Inequities in academic compensation by gender: a follow-up to the National Faculty Survey cohort study. Acad Med 2016;91(8):1068.

13. Eagly AH, Chin JL. Diversity and leadership in a changing world. Am Psychol 2010;65(3):216.

14. Bynum B. Discarded diagnoses. Lancet 2000;356(9241):1615.

15. Drescher J. Out of DSM: depathologizing homosexuality. Behav Sci 2015;5(4):565–75.

16. Metzl JM. The protest psychosis: how schizophrenia became a black disease. Beacon Press: Boston, MA; 2009.

17. Olson KR, Durwood L, DeMeules M, et al. Mental health of transgender children who are supported in their identities. Pediatrics 2016;137(3):e20153223.

18. Hansen H, Braslow J, Rohrbaugh RM. From cultural to structural competency—training psychiatry residents to act on social determinants of health and institutional racism. JAMA Psychiatry 2018;75(2):117–8.

19. Stewart A. Diversity and Inclusion Matter in Continuing Education Efforts. Psychiatr News 2018;53(20):3.

20. American Association of Medical Colleges. Current trends in medical education. Diversity in medical education: facts & figures 2016 2018. Available at: http://www.aamcdiversityfactsandfigures2016.org/report-section/section-3/. Accessed April 10, 2019.

21. Council on Graduate Medical Education. (2005). Minorities in medicine: an ethnic and cultural challenge for physician training - an update 2005. Rockville, MD: U.S. Department of Health and Human Services. Health Resources and Services Administration. Available at: https://www.hrsa.gov/advisorycommittees/bhpradvisory/cogme/Reports/seventeenthrpt.pdf.

22. Marrast LM, Zallman L, Woolhandler S, et al. Minority physicians' role in the care of underserved patients: diversifying the physician workforce may be key in addressing health disparities. JAMA Intern Med 2014;174(2):289–91.

23. Freeman BK, Landry A, Trevino R, et al. Understanding the leaky pipeline: perceived barriers to pursuing a career in medicine or dentistry among underrepresented-in-medicine undergraduate students. Acad Med 2016;91(7):987–93.

24. Dennery P. Training and retaining of underrepresented minority physician scientists–an African-American perspective: NICHD AAP workshop on research in neonatal and perinatal medicine. J Perinatol 2006;26(S2):S46.

25. Lautenberger D, Moses A, Castillo-Page LC. An overview of women full-time medical school faculty of color. Anal Brief 2016;16:1–2. Available at: https://www.aamc.org/download/460728/data/may2016anoverviewofwomenfull-timemedicalschoolfacultyofcolor.pdf.

26. University of Nebraska Medical Center. HIgh School Alliance wins diversity award 2018. Available at: https://www.unmc.edu/news.cfm?match=22375. Accessed April 10, 2019.

27. Nasca TJ, Philibert I, Brigham T, et al. The next GME accreditation system—rationale and benefits. N Engl J Med 2012;366(11):1051–6.

28. The Accreditation Council for Graduate Medical Education and The American Board of Psychiatry and Neurology. The psychiatry milestone project 2015. Available at: https://www.acgme.org/Portals/0/PDFs/Milestones/PsychiatryMilestones.pdf?ver=2015-11-06-120520-753. Accessed April 10, 2019.

29. Bradley SW, Garven JR, Law WW, et al. The impact of chief diversity officers on diverse faculty hiring. National Bureau of Economic Research: Cambridge, MA; 2018.

30. Greenwald AG, McGhee DE, Schwartz JL. Measuring individual differences in implicit cognition: the implicit association test. J Pers Soc Psychol 1998;74(6): 1464.

31. van Ryn M, Hardeman R, Phelan SM, et al. Medical school experiences associated with change in implicit racial bias among 3547 students: a medical student CHANGES study report. J Gen Intern Med 2015;30(12):1748–56.

32. Legault L, Gutsell JN, Inzlicht M. Ironic effects of antiprejudice messages: how motivational interventions can reduce (but also increase) prejudice. Psychol Sci 2011;22(12):1472–7.

33. Association of American Medical Colleges. Leadership development 2018. Available at: https://www.aamc.org/members/leadership/. Accessed April 10, 2019.

34. American Association of Medical Colleges. Healthcare executive diversity and inclusion certificate program 2019. Available at: https://www.aamc.org/initiatives/diversity/portfolios/300950/certificateprogram.html. Accessed April 10, 2019.

35. Drexel University College of Medicine. Executive leadership in academic medicine: fast facts. Available at: https://drexel.edu/medicine/academics/womens-health-and-leadership/elam/about-elam/fast-facts/. Accessed April 10, 2019.

36. Lim RF, Luo JS, Suo S, et al. Diversity initiatives in academic psychiatry: applying cultural competence. Acad Psychiatry 2008;32(4):283–90.

37. Gottlieb AS, Travis EL. Rationale and models for career advancement sponsorship in academic medicine: the time is here; the time is now. Acad Med 2018; 93(11):1620–3.

The Physician's Physician
The Role of the Psychiatrist in Helping Other Physicians and Promoting Wellness

Keisuke Nakagawa, MD*, Peter M. Yellowlees, MBBS, MD

KEYWORDS

- Physician well-being • Wellness • Burnout • Suicide • Depression
- Physician health • Physician well-being committee • Physician health program

KEY POINTS

- Psychiatrists are strategically positioned to serve as leaders in their organizations' efforts to address physician health, including being experts at treating medical colleagues in distress.
- Psychiatrists can serve in several leadership roles at their organizations, including chief wellness officer, chair of the physician well-being committee, and in the state's physician health program.
- Culture change is needed to preserve the health of physicians. It is important to recognize the importance of physician wellness and self-care and adopt the "Quadruple Aim," which includes provider well-being as a core component of the health care system's priorities.
- Psychiatrists need to lead by example in implementing and innovating best practices for supporting physician health in their own practices and by spreading this knowledge to their colleagues.

INTRODUCTION

A recent survey found that nearly two-thirds of US physicians report feeling burnt out, depressed, or both, and it is estimated that approximately 300 to 400 physicians commit suicide every year.[1–3] Although the US health care system and medical culture have always put the patient first, the well-being of physicians has been largely ignored. Although studies have shown that physicians adopt better health care and physical lifestyle practices compared with the general population (regular exercise, less smoking, and less obesity), physicians are also noted to have high rates of mental health concerns.[4,5] At a time when the US health care system faces a critical physician

Disclosure Statement: No disclosures.
Department of Psychiatry and Behavioral Sciences, UC Davis Health, 2230 Stockton Boulevard, Sacramento, CA 95817, USA
* Corresponding author.
E-mail address: drknakagawa@ucdavis.edu

Psychiatr Clin N Am 42 (2019) 473–482
https://doi.org/10.1016/j.psc.2019.05.012
0193-953X/19/© 2019 Elsevier Inc. All rights reserved.

shortage, improving physician health can help to maximize workforce productivity, increase quality of care, and derive more value out of every health care dollar spent.[6,7]

Many positive efforts are already underway by organizations such as the American Medical Association, the American Psychiatric Association, and the Accreditation Council for Graduate Medical Education (ACGME). These include offering online modules, creating toolkits, and mandating resident training on physician well-being, respectively.[8–10] However, significant work remains to adequately address these issues and the medical culture at large. Although physicians receive specialized medical training, their knowledge and expertise does not necessarily enable them to maintain their own personal wellness or model best practices for themselves.

THE PHYSICIAN'S PHYSICIAN: A PSYCHIATRIST'S ROLE
Psychiatrists Have Unique Skills to Treat Physicians

Psychiatrists are in a unique position to serve as the "physician's physician." Most physicians receive very limited training in psychiatry and do not have the skills and knowledge to detect early signs of burnout, depression, addictions, and suicidality in their colleagues or in themselves. This lack of formal training and experience makes it hard for many physicians to take proactive steps to speak to a colleague in distress. Other common causes of delays in addressing colleagues are fear of professional repercussions, damaging relationships, and negatively affecting team dynamics.

Psychiatrists receive substantial training in these skills during residency and throughout their careers. This places psychiatrists in prime position to help their organizations raise awareness and develop effective prevention, detection, and management programs. Historically, psychiatrists have not been proactive enough in promoting the relevance of their skills to help their colleagues and organizations tackle this hidden epidemic.

Psychiatrists Are Well Trained to Treat Very Important Person Physician Patients

Physicians may be challenging to treat. Overidentification, intimidation, and politics can play a significant role in negatively influencing care for the impaired physician who will likely be treated as a VIP. This may lead to deviations from the standard of care that other patients would have received.[11] One of the most common problematic tendencies is for the VIP (physician patient) to influence or dictate their own treatment plans. This leads to a tendency to deviate from standard treatment approaches that the treating physician would have typically made due to fear of upsetting the VIP.[11,12] Excluding physical examinations, delaying drug screens, and ignoring the role of the primary care physician are some common examples of deviations from the standard of care when treating VIPs.

Physicians may also have difficulty being completely honest with their physician patient, resorting to appeasing, or unnecessarily supporting their VIP's demands. This can lead to inappropriate or suboptimal treatments, as both parties lose clinical objectivity. It may be more appropriate and helpful to think of the "VIP" acronym as "Very Influential Patient" or "Very Intimidating Patient" instead of "Very Important Person."[12] This may bring more conscious awareness to the psychosocial traps and biases that can affect even the most cognizant physician.

Another major concern is protecting the privacy of the physician patient. Physician patients will be sensitive to being seen by other staff and colleagues while seeking care, and it is not uncommon for appointments to be scheduled outside of regular clinic hours. Physician patients often prefer to be referred outside of their practice network and pay cash to avoid having their employer or insurer having any record of their visits. Some physician patients also expect priority treatment such as being able to call their physician's cell phone directly.[11] It can be helpful to offer these, but it is critical to set clear limits.

Informal Consults: a Supportive Colleague Just One Phone Call Away

Within a health system or clinical network, psychiatrists can serve to help support and identify colleagues at risk for depression, burnout, and suicide. Physicians struggling with depression and burnout may try to hide their symptoms from colleagues for fear of professional repercussions, stigma, and judgment. Many will also be in self-denial and try to "power through" their struggle as other obstacles they have had to overcome in their life. Having a colleague who they can trust, talk to, and confide in can be one of the most effective first-line defenses. One of the most effective ways for organizations to identify struggling physicians is creating an informal referral network that includes a psychiatrist who is available to provide information and anonymous consultations.

BEST PRACTICES FOR ADDRESSING IMPAIRED PHYSICIANS AND PROMOTING WELLNESS

A large proportion of physicians report experiencing at least one symptom of burnout.[13] Many physicians have colleagues who are burnt out but are unaware of the fact and may hesitate to address such colleagues when they notice warning signs, because they receive little to no training on how to do so effectively. Having education on well-being for all physicians, and making self-care part of the culture of health care, are likely effective responses.

A Culture of Wellness as the First Defense

A clear message and acknowledgment of the impact of burnout from leadership such as the Chief Executive Officer and Chief Wellness Officer (CWO) are important first steps to promoting a culture of wellness across the organization, as long as this is done in a manner that does not blame physicians or make it seem that they are the problem. In reality, current evidence suggests that 80% of burnout is caused by administrative and systems issues, not by a lack of resilience from individual physicians. Creating open forums for staff to learn about wellness strategies and discuss burnout issues elevate the awareness of staff across the entire organization as a valuable first-line defense.[11] It is also important to create systems and processes such as anonymous hotlines, well-being committees, and reporting protocols that reduce the barrier to self-reporting or reporting a colleague (**Box 1**).

Addressing Impaired Physicians, Substance Abuse, and Addiction

Risk factors and warning signs for suicide are not different for physicians compared with the general public.[14] Educating staff on these warning signs is a critical first step to prevention, early identification, and management of burnt out physicians at risk for suicide.

It is important for colleagues to take immediate action if they notice changes in a colleague. Expressing concern for the individual, asking about their well-being, or suggesting that they speak to a mental health professional can be a critical first step to helping the individual.[11] Regularly reinforcing these points with the team at staff meetings, one-on-one sessions, and continuing medical education coursework can increase awareness and reduce the stigma that is one of the most common causes for delayed action by colleagues.

Box 1
Ten best practices for promoting wellness and addressing physician burnout

Leadership. Communicate a clear vision and plan for supporting wellness efforts. Acknowledge burnout issues and reinforce leadership's commitment to addressing them.

Well-Being Committee. Start a physician well-being committee and assign wellness champions across departments and employment levels.

Performance Metrics. Align staff performance metrics with wellness activities and objectives.

Quality Metrics. Incorporate wellness-oriented metrics as part of the organization's quality measures.

Annual Survey. Distribute an annual wellness survey to establish a concrete baseline and solicit feedback.

Interventions. Launch pilot programs based on feedback and ideas.

Data Collection. Use follow-up surveys and focus groups to measure progress and impact with quantitative and qualitative data.

Refinement. Use survey data and feedback to refine interventions and iterate on improvements. Scale successful interventions to increase impact and expand outreach.

Reinforcement. Meet regularly with leaders and staff to discuss progress, data, and interventions to promote wellness.

Systems. Establish processes to systematize key functions that reduce the barriers to getting help. Examples include anonymous self-reporting hotlines, processes for reporting colleagues, and well-being committees.

Data from American Medical Association (AMA), STEPS Forward™. Preventing Physician Burnout: improve patient satisfaction, quality outcomes and provider recruitment and retention; 2018; and Yellowlees PM. Physician suicide: cases and commentaries, 1st edition. Washington, DC: American Psychiatric Association Publishing; 2019.

It is vital to be educated on the difference between having a disorder, such as depression, and a disability or an impairment. The latter may cause work-related difficulties and require reporting through appropriate internal or external channels, potentially to a Physician Health Program, or occasionally directly to Medical Boards. Most physician patients with a psychiatric- or substance-related problem have an illness and are not impaired for work in any functional way, and they should be treated clinically and reassured that no reporting is necessary.

ORGANIZATIONAL LEADERSHIP ROLES FOR PSYCHIATRISTS TO CHAMPION PHYSICIAN WELL-BEING

Psychiatrists can play an instrumental role in driving a culture of physician well-being for their organizations. In 2017, the ACGME started requiring all accredited residency and fellowship programs "to address well-being more directly and comprehensively" (Section VI of Common Program Requirements).[10,15] This is an opportunity for psychiatrists to help craft policies, guidelines, and programs that fulfill these new requirements.

Psychiatrists can increasingly serve as valuable leaders and contributors to every organization by serving as CWO, chairing or being a member of a physician well-being committee, or working with a statewide physician health program (PHP). A description of each role is provided in more detail below summarizing key responsibilities, required skills, process for getting involved, and the kind of impact one can make in an organization by serving in such roles. These roles also offer opportunities for professional development and career enrichment for psychiatrists looking to expand the scope of their practice, engage in physician leadership, and leverage their clinical expertise to shape policies at the local and national levels.

Chair or Member of Physician Well-Being Committee

Physician well-being committees involve volunteer physicians at a hospital or health system and fulfill the 2001 mandate from the Joint Commission that requires accredited health care organizations to implement "a process to identify and manage matters of individual health for licensed independent practitioners which is separate from actions taken for disciplinary purposes." This has tended to comprise a physician well-being committee.[16,17]

The functions and practices of physician well-being committees vary significantly. Most committees focus on identification, assessment, and referral of impaired physicians to the State PHP, which takes care of the monitoring and management of the physician until they are deemed safe to return to practice. Both systems are meant to be nonpunitive and offer a safe, recovery process that does not involve the State Medical Board or de-licensing.

Physician well-being committees are good career entry points for physicians interested in getting more involved in physician health issues. Psychiatrists are well-positioned to chair these committees, given their expertise in mental health. Serving on these committees can offer a unique perspective on addiction and mental health issues, because the committee sits at the intersection of clinical practice, policy, and institutional leadership and management.

Chief Wellness Officer

CWOs are new executive level positions that often set the long-term vision, strategy, and implementation of wellness for the organization. Among the 168 LCME-accredited medical schools and 400 major teaching hospitals in North America, as of November 2018, 18 had appointed CWOs, only 2 of whom were psychiatrists.

CWOs require many different skillsets, although the addition of strong clinical expertise in mental health would seem to be most useful, making psychiatrists well positioned to fill these roles. A CWO typically manages a multidisciplinary team that spans the entire organization, has experience setting long-term vision and strategies, as well as developing shorter-term goals focused on implementation of organizational changes and well-being initiatives. CWOs have the potential to impact an organization's culture, productivity, and success. Workforce training and retention can be one of the most significant drivers of cost for any organization. Lost productivity due to physician burnout and depression is costly, leading to decreased patient volume, increased stress on other physicians who need to cover, and negative impact on quality of care as a consequence. One study calculated that the US health system incurs $3.4 billion in annual costs due to physician burnout, and a study conducted at Stanford University estimated the annual cost to their health system to be in the range of $8 million to $28 million.[6,18,19] Therefore, supporting a culture where physicians and staff can find more fulfillment, meaning, and joy in their work every day can have a significant impact on the long-term success of an organization.

State Physician Health Programs

PHPs are nonpunitive and nondisciplinary state-run programs that help physicians address their addictions and mental health conditions, recover, and create a safe, structured, and accountable plan to return to practice.

PHPs are composed of a medical director and a few full-time or part-time staff who are often psychiatrists or addiction specialists, and they are employed by the state running the PHP. It is important to note that their services are not generally free and have to be paid by physicians using them. This can cause a professional dilemma for impaired physicians, because complying with the PHPs' program may be a requirement to avoid being reported to the state medical board while they recover. However, the PHPs offer a valuable service for recovering physicians, and follow-up studies have shown that up to 80% of physicians with substance use disorders, including psychiatrists, return to practice within 5 years.[20,21]

TRAINING AND ORGANIZATIONAL CAPACITY BUILDING

There are 3 major training requirements: first, the need for self-care for all physicians; second, educational programs for physicians who wish to treat other physicians; third, institutional and departmental promotion and education of a culture of wellness. With new requirements set by ACGME for integrating physician health education in all residency programs starting in 2017, a more streamlined curriculum to assist physicians with their own self-care would be valuable to provide a standardized baseline of knowledge and skills for all physicians.[15,22]

Training in self-care and well-being is likely to be most effective when it is incorporated throughout the course of the physician's training starting in medical school. Most medical schools have resources available, including wellness counselors and academic advisors. This presents a great opportunity for psychiatry to play a more integral role in the medical school curriculum and throughout the training pipeline from medical school, to residency, to clinical practice. A comprehensive curriculum for self-care and well-being would cover a range of topics including resilience, regular participation in process-oriented reflective small groups, mindfulness training, and interpersonal skills development (**Box 2**).

Box 2
Key elements of comprehensive curriculum on physician self-care and well-being

Small Groups. Regular participation in process-oriented reflective small groups.

Networking and Relationships. Teach ways to strengthen professional and social relationships and how to network widely and appropriately. Specific skill development in interpersonal professional relationships.

Simulations, Multimedia, and Experiential Training. Media training, combined with experiential training using multiple communications technologies with patients and colleagues.

Mentorship. Mentoring and mentee supervision opportunities throughout medical school and residency.

Self-Reflection. Content and discussion of personal identity development and transformation, the interaction between burnout and physician health, empathy, compassion, and how to become reflective practitioners.

Mindfulness and Resilience Training. Active participation and learning about resilience, mindfulness, exercise, nutrition, and relationships.

Psychiatry for Physicians. Content on the specific psychiatric, substance abuse, and personality disorders that affect physicians and how to recognize and treat them in any physician, including the individual themselves.

Leadership and Skills Training. Modules and discussion groups on leadership, financial, and business skills.

Systems Training. Learning about organizational systems and the interactions that occur within them and an understanding of institutional awareness and resources that can be used to change institutions.

Adapting to Practice Changes. Decision-making and clinical reasoning that takes into account future changes in medicine and technology such as the need for physicians to analyze large datasets and translate to patients.

Data from Yellowlees PM. Physician suicide: cases and commentaries, 1st edition. Washington, DC: American Psychiatric Association Publishing; 2019.

Psychiatrists serving in organizational leadership capacities are strategically positioned to advocate for more exposure to their specialty during the critical period where students are assessing their careers and residency options.

No formal training program exists outside of psychiatry residency for physicians to be trained to manage physician health issues. Many physicians gain experience and knowledge by serving on committees or by treating physicians as patients. Although receiving "on-the-job" training such as this can be effective, there is wide variation in exposure and experience, and specialist training programs in this area are sorely needed.

EMBRACING CULTURAL EVOLUTION

In 2014, the Institute for Healthcare Improvement revised their original Triple Aim framework to include "Joy in Work" to make it the "Quadruple Aim."[23,24] Physicians and physicians-in-training need to be empowered to protect their health and well-being just as much as they are taught to put the patient's needs first. They both do not need to be at odds if the culture and practices evolve to protect both patients and physicians.

"It is unprofessional not to look after yourself," is a message that is rarely taught and needs to be emphasized more in the future. We need to teach a broad scope of professionalism beyond attire, appearance, timeliness, and bedside manners. The Hippocratic Oath is full of values that protect the patient's rights, but there is no mention of how physicians need to treat themselves. Many medical schools have final year students modify this oath annually and it is to be hoped that such modifications will increasingly include the importance of self-care as a professional attribute.

Psychiatrists Leading Health Care's Workforce into the Future

The country's health care workforce is rapidly changing with a new generation of physicians entering clinical practice and the baby boomer generation of physicians set to retire. Technologies such as telemedicine and smartphones are enabling more flexible and mobile work arrangements. Psychiatrists can lead a process in adapting to these new changes and evolve their practices accordingly. Today's culture and work environments need to change rapidly to support the values and work-life equilibria sought by the Millennial generation. The changes in residency applications to various specialties are indicators of the shift in workforce preferences with increasing applications to "lifestyle" specialties such as dermatology and emergency medicine. Although Millennials are often described as "high maintenance" or "entitled," they are also known to prioritize family, friends, and hobbies, making them more resilient to burnout and better at self-care than previous generations.[11,25,26] Millennials are responding to the pressures of modern medicine more effectively than previous generations of physicians, and the medical culture will have to change to take into account the needs of this upcoming generation of physicians.

Technology also plays an undeniable role in physician burnout. Electronic medical records, increased administrative workloads, and increasing emphasis on laboratories, evidence, and data analysis will inevitably affect the way physicians practice medicine and how much joy and meaning they can find in their daily practice.[27,28] How will physicians increase meaning and joy through patient care while integrating more data and technology into their clinical workflows? These are the difficult questions that need to be studied to guide the profession toward a more fulfilling practice in the future. Innovations in telemedicine, smartphones, and web-based technologies create new opportunities for physicians to adopt a more hybrid approach to their practice that integrates virtual care more into their daily practice. Psychiatrists have opportunities to shape the future practice of medicine, using their understanding of cognition and mental processes to improve workflows by designing innovative user experiences and products.

LEADING BY EXAMPLE: MODELING SELF-CARE

It is important to remember that psychiatrists are also vulnerable to burnout and depression although rates are low compared with other specialties.[28] Although we focus on opportunities to lead and support physician health in communities, we must lead by example as individuals and as a specialty. During residency, psychiatrists learn the professional demands of clinical practice, and this is a critical time to teach best practices on wellness and self-care to all psychiatric residents. Psychiatrists' everyday actions and behaviors can have the most impact on their colleagues and health systems.

From a research perspective, psychiatrists have the opportunity to advance their understanding of physician health and well-being through research, advocacy, and clinical excellence. Very few studies have evaluated the design, implementation, and effectiveness of physician health programs such as physician well-being committees or state PHPs, and self-care education programs need to be evaluated as they are introduced. Data are critical to understand what is working and what is not working and for the community to share best practices that lead to measurable outcomes. The growing physician health problem opens the door for new research opportunities and advocacy efforts that are well-suited for psychiatrists to lead.

SUMMARY

Increasing interest in physician health and well-being offers a unique opportunity for psychiatrists to elevate their profession's visibility and affect the organizational and national levels. The country's health care spending is on an unsustainable trajectory, while the physician shortage problem will only get worse as more physicians retire. Lost productivity due to physician burnout, depression, and addiction is no longer just a physician wellness issue, but it has become a national policy issue. For the health care system to gain more value out of every health care dollar, maintaining a healthy, productive physician workforce is absolutely critical.

Despite organized efforts to tackle this problem as state PHPs and the Joint Commission's mandate of implementing physician well-being committees, the culture and everyday practice of medicine still lags behind. There is an opportunity for psychiatrists to serve in numerous roles to help drive cultural change and become leaders at the organizational, regional, and national levels. Designing and implementing effective physician well-being programs requires experienced mental health professionals to provide guidance and expertise to maximize returns on these investments, while improving patient care and physician well-being.

REFERENCES

1. Peckham C. Medscape national physician burnout & depression report 2018 2018. Medscape. Available at: https://www.medscape.com/slideshow/2018-lifestyle-burnout-depression-6009235. Accessed August 22, 2018.
2. Center C, Davis M, Detre T, et al. Confronting depression and suicide in physicians: a consensus statement. JAMA 2003;289(23):3161–6.
3. Association of American Medical Colleges. Applicants and matriculants data - FACTS: applicants, matriculants, enrollment, graduates, MD/PhD, and residency applicants data - data and analysis - AAMC. Applicants and matriculants data. Available at: https://www.aamc.org/data/facts/applicantmatriculant/. Accessed August 23, 2018.
4. Helfand BKI, Mukamal KJ. Healthcare and lifestyle practices of healthcare workers: do healthcare workers practice what they preach? JAMA Intern Med 2013;173(3):242–4.
5. Compton MT, Frank E. Mental health concerns among Canadian physicians: results from the 2007-2008 Canadian Physician Health Study. ComprPsychiatry 2011;52(5):542–7.
6. Berg S. At Stanford, physician burnout costs at least $7.75 million a year. AMA Wire. 2017. Available at: https://wire.ama-assn.org/life-career/stanford-physician-burnout-costs-least-775-million-year. Accessed August 23, 2018.
7. Shanafelt T, Goh J, Sinsky C. The business case for investing in physician well-being. JAMA Intern Med 2017;177(12):1826–32.
8. Linzer M, Guzman-Corrales L, Poplau S. Preventing physician Burnout - STEPS forward.AMA | STEPS forward. Available at: https://www.stepsforward.org/modules/physician-burnout. Accessed August 23, 2018.
9. Goldman ML, Bernstein C, Chilton J, et al. Toolkit for well-being ambassadors: a manual - a guide for psychiatrists to improve physician well-being and reduce physician burnout at their institutions. 2017. Available at: https://www.psychiatry.org/psychiatrists/practice/well-being-and-burnout/well-being-resources. Accessed August 23, 2018.
10. Accreditation Council for Graduate Medical Education (ACGME). Improving physician well-being, restoring meaning in medicine. 2018. ACGME.Available at: https://www.acgme.org/What-We-Do/Initiatives/Physician-Well-Being. Accessed August 23, 2018.
11. Yellowlees PM. Physician suicide: cases and commentaries. 1st edition. Washington, DC: American Psychiatric Association Publishing; 2019.
12. Alfandre D, Clever S, Farber NJ, et al. Caring for 'very important patients'–ethical dilemmas and suggestions for practical management. Am J Med 2016;129(2):143–7.
13. Shanafelt TD, Hasan O, Dyrbye LN, et al. Changes in Burnout and satisfaction with work-life balance in physicians and the general US working population between 2011 and 2014. MayoClin Proc 2015;90(12):1600–13.
14. Preventing physician distress and suicide. Available at: https://edhub.ama-assn.org/steps-forward/module/2702599. Accessed December 28, 2018.
15. Accreditation Council for Graduate Medical Education (ACGME). ACGME common program requirements section VI with background and intent 2017. Available at: https://www.acgme.org/What-We-Do/Accreditation/Common-Program-Requirements. Accessed August 23, 2018.
16. CMA Legal Counsel and California Public, Protection and Physician Health. 5177 guidelines for physician well-being committees policies and procedures 2013.

Available at: https://www.csam-asam.org/sites/default/files/5177_oncall.pdf. Accessed August 8, 2013.

17. Joint commission requirement - MS.11.01.01. Available at: http://www.massmed.org/Physician_Health_Services/Joint_Commission/Joint_Commission_Requirement_-_MS_11_01_01/#.W375GugzpEY. Accessed August 23, 2018.

18. Goh J, Shasha Han MS, Shanafelt TD, et al. An economic evaluation of the cost of physician burnout in the United States. In: Abstract book. 2017. p. 102. San Francisco (CA): American Conference on Physician Health (ACPH); 2017. Available at: https://med.stanford.edu/content/dam/sm/CME/documents/brochures/2017/ACPH-Abstract-Book-FULL.pdf.

19. Hamidi MS, Bohman B, Sandborg C, et al. The economic cost of physician turnover attributable to burnout. In: Abstract book. 2017. p. 35. San Francisco (CA): American Conference on Physician Health (ACPH); 2017.

20. DuPont RL, McLellan AT, Carr G, et al. How are addicted physicians treated? A national survey of Physician Health Programs. J SubstAbuse Treat 2009; 37(1):1–7.

21. Yellowlees PM, Campbell MD, Rose JS, et al. Psychiatrists with substance use disorders: positive treatment outcomes from physician health programs. Psychiatr Serv 2014;65(12):1492–5.

22. White S. ACGME launches resources webpage for resident and faculty well-being. The DO 2018. Available at: https://thedo.osteopathic.org/2018/03/acgme-launches-resources-webpage-resident-faculty-well/. Accessed August 23, 2018.

23. Bodenheimer T, Sinsky C. From triple to quadruple aim: care of the patient requires care of the provider. Ann Fam Med 2014;12(6):573–6.

24. Feeley D. The triple aim or the quadruple aim? Four points to help set your strategy. IHIImprov Blog. 2017. Available at: http://www.ihi.org/communities/blogs/the-triple-aim-or-the-quadruple-aim-four-points-to-help-set-your-strategy. Accessed August 23, 2018.

25. Landrum S. Millennials to be the most high-maintenance in the workplace. Forbes 2018. Available at: https://www.forbes.com/sites/sarahlandrum/2018/01/12/millennials-to-be-the-most-high-maintenance-in-the-workplace/. Accessed August 23, 2018.

26. Hershatter A, Epstein M. Millennials and the world of work: an organization and management perspective. J Bus Psychol 2010;25(2):211–23.

27. Sinsky C, Colligan L, Li L, et al. Allocation of physician time in ambulatory practice: a time and motion study in 4 specialties. Ann Intern Med 2016;165(11): 753–60.

28. Arndt BG, Beasley JW, Watkinson MD, et al. Tethered to the EHR: primary care physician workload assessment using EHRevent log data and time-motion observations. Ann Fam Med 2017;15(5):419–26.

Social Media Skills for Professional Development in Psychiatry and Medicine

Howard Y. Liu, MD[a],*, Eugene V. Beresin, MD, MA[b],
Margaret S. Chisolm, MD[c]

KEYWORDS

- Social media • Twitter • Networking • Career development • Professionalism
- Technology • Digital health • e-health

KEY POINTS

- Twitter is a useful social media platform to facilitate professional development and advocacy.
- Social media can help psychiatrists develop a professional brand.
- Networking is one of the great advantages of social media.
- Several organizations, journals, and specialty societies are using Twitter to enhance member engagement and interest in resources/articles.
- Psychiatrists should observe standards of digital citizenship and professionalism when using social media.

INTRODUCTION

Social media refers to online tools that allow swift sharing of content among users.[1] Common platforms in the United States include YouTube, Facebook, Instagram, Pinterest, Snapchat, LinkedIn, Twitter, and WhatsApp (**Table 1**).[2] According to a report from the Pew Research Center, a typical American uses 3 social media platforms regularly, and social media use increases with each generation. Social media use is reported by 88% of Americans aged 18 to 29 years, 78% of Americans aged 30 to 49 years, 64% of Americans aged 50 to 64 years, and 37% of Americans aged 65 years and older.[2] Social media use is becoming increasingly common in health care

Disclosure Statement: No disclosures for any of the authors.
[a] Department of Psychiatry, University of Nebraska Medical Center, 985575 Nebraska Medical Center, Omaha, NE 68198-5575, USA; [b] Harvard Medical School, Massachusetts General Hospital One Bowdoin Square, 9th Floor, Boston, MA 02114, USA; [c] Johns Hopkins Medicine, 5300 Alpha Commons Drive, Baltimore, MD 21224, USA
* Corresponding author.
E-mail address: hyliu@unmc.edu
; @DrHowardLiu (H.Y.L.); @GeneBeresinMD (E.V.B.); @whole_patients (M.S.C.)

Psychiatr Clin N Am 42 (2019) 483–492
https://doi.org/10.1016/j.psc.2019.05.004
0193-953X/19/© 2019 The Authors. Published by Elsevier Inc. This is an open access article under the CC BY-NC-ND license (http://creativecommons.org/licenses/by-nc-nd/4.0/).

Table 1
Comparison of popular social media platforms and utility for psychiatrists

Platform	User Base (% of US Adults in 2018)	Advantages for Psychiatry Professional Use	Disadvantages for Psychiatry Professional Use
YouTube	73%	Videos, high user base	Restricted to video content
Facebook	68%	Photos, videos, high user base	Professionalism boundaries can be harder to maintain, as many use the platform for personal life
Instagram	35%	Posts with a primary visual media—photos, videos with less text	Psychiatry typically is less image based than a field such as pathology or surgery
Pinterest	29%	Collecting quotes and ideas for talks	Limited psychiatric and medical organizations on the platform
Snapchat	27%	High user base, particularly with Millennials and Generation Z	Pictures and messages disappear, considered a more informal platform
LinkedIn	25%	Posting articles, jobs, discussion groups	Conversations tend to be slower and more measured
Twitter	24%	Many psychiatric organizations and physicians are on the platform	Fewer Generation Z and Millennials on the platform

Data from Smith A, Anderson M. Social media Use in 2018. Pew Research Center. 2018; Accessed December 15, 2018. Available at: https://urldefense.proofpoint.com/v2/url?u=https-3A__www.pewinternet.org_2018_03_01_social-2Dmedia-2Duse-2Din-2D2018_&d=DwIGaQ&c=ZukO2flan9e5E9v43wuy1w&r=IVuPPozG-Flvt_KR7aGheQ&m=HlE5njZvRCaRfEqF5jtxj2ei-CRUgD0wEjutBNdijH8&s=NP1Bhr9OhuCy_0hpAdKFVWQ4m7vfzSuARMGrIGRdGgk&e=

and academia, with major organizations such as the American Medical Association and the Council of Residency Directors developing professionalism guidelines for members.[3] The proliferation of higher education on Twitter has been deemed "Academic Twitter" to denote the community of scholars actively engaged on social media.[4] Indeed, patients are also becoming more empowered and have increasing expectations to gather information and interact with their physicians and psychiatrists electronically as equals.[5]

The field of psychiatry is exploring competencies in social media ranging from patient care to interpersonal and communication skills.[6] In this article, the authors focus on the use of Twitter for professional development in psychiatry. The same principles apply to other branches of medicine, as has been well described by other social media pioneers in surgery, medical oncology, emergency medicine, etc.[7–10] As a field, psychiatry translates well to text-based platforms such as Twitter with its emphasis on interviews and the humanities. In addition, the increasing number of psychiatrists, psychiatric organizations, psychiatric journals, and medical organizations on Twitter render it a highly useful platform for professional development.

USING TWITTER FOR PROFESSIONAL DEVELOPMENT

This article explores how to use Twitter to create a professional brand as a psychiatrist. It will not focus on the personal use of Twitter for recreation or political advocacy as a private citizen. Social media can be a powerful medium to amplify professional work, but it must be balanced with sponsoring and promoting the work of others. Twitter is fundamentally an inclusive platform, as any individual can open an account and voice their opinions regardless of academic rank or seniority in the standard medical hierarchy.[7] Here are a few principles to observe:

- Brevity: as Shakespeare once stated, "brevity is the soul of wit." Twitter is a microblogging platform that limits posts to 280 characters. It takes practice for psychiatrists who are often accustomed to longer conversations to compress their thoughts into brief posts.
- Restraint: on all social media platforms, psychiatrists should expect to encounter online debates. Occasionally, these debates can grow heated and devolve into ad hominem attacks. The authors advise to limit these interactions and avoid "feeding the trolls." With contemporary topics from gun violence to immigration policy blurring the line between personal and professional, it is up to each psychiatrist and their employer to determine where to draw that line.
- Generativity: Twitter tracks how many individuals a user follows and how many individuals follow that user. It is advisable to follow individuals and organizations that one admires or are seeking to promote. Although it is acceptable to share one's own publications or promotions, this may be viewed as narcissistic if the great majority of posts are self-congratulatory. A good rule of thumb is to use a 1:10 or 1:20 ratio of "posts that reflect my accomplishments" to "posts that lift up others in the field." Retweeting others (the process of forwarding the posts of other users) is considered good social media etiquette, and adding a positive comment about a post goes even further.

CREATING A PROFESSIONAL TWITTER PROFILE

The first step when starting on Twitter is to create a high-impact professional profile.
The profile should accomplish several tasks: increase the psychiatrist's credibility, align them with health care organizations, illustrate areas of professional expertise or passion, and offer a brief biography. Components of a strong professional profile include the following:

- Logical Twitter handle[11]: the Twitter handle is the name that others use to identify the user on social media. Because Twitter has a global following, there may very well be more than one individual with a psychiatrist's first and last name. One tip is to add "Dr" to the beginning or "MD" at the end of one's first and last name. Thus, Jane Doe could be "DrJaneDoe" or "JaneDoeMD." If the screen name is taken, it is acceptable to add numbers to the end (ie, "JaneDoeMD3"), and the rest of the profile will help colleagues identify the correct individual.
- Professional profile photo: typically, this would be a professional head shot. For a more irreverent profile, psychiatrists can use applications such as Bitmoji to create a cartoon avatar. However, social media users often use the profile picture to ensure that they are following the correct individual, so the profile photo should help identify the psychiatrist.
- Interesting header photo: a banner at the top of the profile that allows a user to include a quote, a photo, a logo, or another visual symbol. For professional profiles, users may want to consult their public relations office before using official organizational logos or photos, as there may be some restrictions on branding.
- Bio including organizations and hashtags: listing the psychiatrist's employer, organizations with a special significance to the psychiatrist, and topics of importance will help like-minded individuals to locate the psychiatrist on social

media. Hashtags refer to words preceded by the "#", same that are used to search for topics and organize conversations. They are commonly used at national conferences to organize all of the posts or "tweets" into one stream that can concentrate the conversation and allow it to be measured or tracked. For example, if a psychiatrist was a clinical educator, they might list #meded in their profile. See **Table 2** for a list of common organizations, journals, and clinical specialty societies on Twitter.

- Website: users can include a link to a personal or professional Website.
- Location: this allows the user to list their city, state, and country or keep it anonymous.

Table 2
Psychiatric educational organizations, research agencies, journals, and specialty societies

Organization	Twitter Handle	Followers
Educational Organizations		
Association of American Medical Colleges (AAMC)	@AAMCToday	47,500
Accreditation Council for Graduate Medical Education (ACGME)	@acgme	4964
Harvard Macy Institute	@harvardmacy	4163
Research Agencies		
National Institute of Mental Health (NIMH)	@NIMHgov	1.15M
National Institutes of Health (NIH)	@NIH	878,000
National Institute on Drug Abuse (NIDA)	@NIDAnews	45,500
Substance Abuse and Mental Health Services Administration (SAMHSA)	@samhsagov	87,100
Journals		
The New England Journal of Medicine (NEJM)	@NEJM	548,800
The Journal of the American Medical Association (JAMA)	@JAMA_current	275,300
The Journal of the American Medical Association Psychiatry (JAMA Psychiatry)	@JAMAPsych	22,100
The Journal of Clinical Psychiatry	@JClinPsychiatry	20,700
Elsevier Psychiatry (collates all psych journals from this publisher)	@els_psychiatry	8519
The American Journal of Psychiatry	@AmJPsychiatry	1778
The Journal of the American Academy of Child & Adolescent Psychiatry (JAACAP)	@JAACAP	788
Academic Psychiatry	@AcadPsychiatry	431
Psychiatry Specialty Organizations		
American Psychiatric Association (APA)	@APAPsychiatric	90,300
American Society of Addiction Medicine (ASAM)	@ASAMorg	14,800
American Academy of Child & Adolescent Psychiatry (AACAP)	@AACAP	12,500
American Academy of Addiction Psychiatry (AAAP)	@AAAP1985	4090
American Association For Geriatric Psychiatry (AAGP)	@GeriPsyc	1347

Note, this is a sample in each category and is not meant to be inclusive. Followers were assessed on December 15, 2018 and will likely change by date of publication.
Data from Twitter. Available at: https://twitter.com/. Accessed Dec 15, 2018.

- Pinned tweet: Twitter currently allows users to keep one post constantly at the top of their profile page. This is an opportunity to showcase a message that illustrates the user's philosophy, values, sense of humor, etc. A common practice is to analyze a user's tweets using Twitter analytics and to pin a popular post to one's profile.

NETWORKING ON SOCIAL MEDIA

One of the primary benefits of social media is the ability to network with colleagues rapidly and across disciplines. When attending a national conference, tweeting to the conference hashtag enables other attendees to see your profile and vice versa. This allows psychiatrists to rapidly identify other psychiatrists, mental health advocates, and thought leaders at a conference. This also permits psychiatrist to directly interact with speakers and even celebrities and political figures either publicly by replying to or retweeting their message or by sending them a private Direct Message to invite future collaboration. Because most users do not include their e-mail addresses in their profiles, direct messaging is a common way to request an e-mail address for further dialogue.

If a psychiatrist is mentoring a trainee or a colleague, social media can also be used to promote that individual's career; this can be done by sharing or retweeting the mentee's paper, announcing the colleague's promotion or award, and consistently interacting with the colleague's social media messages to show support. The more followers that a psychiatrist or organization has, the more powerful the amplifying effect of retweeting a mentee's tweet is. For example, if a mentoring psychiatrist has 5000 followers, then the retweet will generate far more engagements than if a mentoring psychiatrist has 50 followers.

Between conferences, the strategic and consistent use of hashtags (see **Table 3** for definition) helps the psychiatrist to identify others who share similar professional interests. For example, medical educators frequently include the hashtag #meded on their tweets to allow other educators to find them. Addiction Medicine providers or Addiction Psychiatrists could include the hashtags #addiction or #substanceuse on their tweets. And psychiatrists working in the public sector to decrease stigma might use the hashtags #MentalHealthMatters or #MentalHealthAwareness. Finally, users can create their own hashtags but should search for them first on Twitter to ensure that they are not already used by another organization or do not have another connotation.

SOCIAL MEDIA FOR EDUCATION AND RESEARCH

Social media can be a catalyst for academic psychiatrists for education and research. Twitter can be used as a tool for medical educators in many ways. A teacher could enroll students on Twitter and then use a Twitter hashtag to create an interactive conversation displayed live for students to respond to questions in real time.[12] There is emerging evidence of its use as a pedagogical tool to increase student engagement with staff, peers, and course content where the use of Twitter enabled greater accessibility to staff.[13] It can also be a forum to find collaborators for academic projects such as national presentations, peer-reviewed publications, and grants. Following journals (see **Table 2**) and educational organizations on Twitter also helps psychiatric educators stay abreast of the latest developments in the field.

For researchers, there are increasing calls for science to move beyond laboratories and into the public domain for broader dissemination. There is a strong scientific community on social media, but it is not evenly distributed. A recent study found that social, computer and information scientists are overrepresented on Twitter, whereas

Table 3 Twitter glossary	
Term	**Definition**
Analytics	A built in dashboard where users can analyze the impact of each tweet including the engagement and provide demographic and topical interests of your followers.
Bio	A brief description of the user.
Block	Choosing to stop another user from following you or your tweets. Users will not be notified if a blocked user mentions them in a tweet.
Direct Message (DM)	Sending a private message to a Twitter user that is not visible to others on Twitter.
Engagement	Total number of times a user interacted with a tweet including retweets, replies, follows, likes, links, etc.
Follow	Signing up to view tweets from another user. The standard following limit is currently up to 5000 accounts until the user surpasses a certain number of followers.
Follower	Another user who follows your account.
Handle	The user's name on Twitter that begins with an @ symbol (eg, @DrJaneDoe).
Hashtag (#)	Symbol used to group conversations and topics on Twitter. The # symbol precedes the word (eg, #psychiatry).
Home	A timeline that continually updates with content from accounts you have chosen to follow.
Impressions	Number of times users saw a tweet on Twitter. Along with engagements, one of the metrics that are used to determine the dissemination of a tweet.
Like	A heart symbol that a user can click to show support for a tweet. Likes are visible to other Twitter users when they visit your profile, and this should be noted for a professional Twitter profile.
Mention	When another user includes your Twitter handle in their post.
Mute	Removing a user's tweets from your Twitter home. This does not unfollow an individual and they are not notified.
Notifications	Alerts that update a user when another individual has interacted with your tweet. This includes a Like, Retweet, or Mention.
Profile	A user's bio and pinned tweet and a list of all of the user's tweets starting with the most recent one.
Retweet (RT)	Forwarding on another user's tweet to your followers.
Tweet	A message or post that can be up to 280 characters long. It can include text, photos, or videos.
Tweeting	The process of posting a message or tweet.

Data from Twitter Help Center. Using Twitter. Available at: https://help.twitter.com/en/using-twitter. Accessed April 21, 2019.

mathematical, life and physical scientists are underrepresented.[14] The same study suggested that although there was still a gender disparity, there was less of a disparity on Twitter than in traditional scientific publications. The investigators found that the female to male ratio was 0.629 on Twitter compared with 0.428 for traditional scientific publications in the United States.[14] Another study found that scientists with less than 1000 followers were mostly read by fellow scientists, but if they surpassed 1000 followers, then their followers became more diverse and included more nonscientists.[15] This illustrates the potential that avid Twitter use can lead to greater dissemination of science to policy makers, advocates, patients, etc.

Finally, germane to both psychiatric education and research is the relatively new field called altmetrics, which measures the dissemination and potential impact of individual peer-reviewed journal articles and alternative academic products (eg, webinars, instructional videos, blogs) through online metrics.[16] These alternative metrics summarize how research is shared and discussed online and complement traditional citation-based metrics, such as the journal impact factor and h-index.[16] One definition used by Maggio and colleagues[17] is that altmetrics are "web-based metrics for the impact of scholarly material, with an emphasis on social media outlets as sources of data." In an analysis of 2486 articles related to health profession education, blogging was associated with the greatest increase in citations (13%), whereas tweets only increased citations by 1.2%.[16] However, Twitter is noted to be popular among scholars and journals and a forum for frequent discussions about scholarly work.[17] For example, one analysis suggests that a greater number of Twitter mentions is associated with more citations in the American Journal of Psychiatry (see **Table 2** for a list of medical and psychiatric journals on Twitter).[18] Further research is needed, as there are complicating factors such as whether an article's full text was publicly accessible. Also, a high number of altmetric events does not necessarily indicate quality but merely quantifies attention—both positive or negative.[17] Despite these limitations, scholars are encouraging principal investigators to include altmetrics on their curriculum vitae as a measure of public engagement and outreach.[19] And there may be an even greater impact for strategic use of social media by women physicians who can leverage online networks to overcome traditional barriers to advancement in academic health centers.[20] In sum, a psychiatrist or physician seeking to increase readership of a recently published journal article could consider amplifying its dissemination via a blog and social media and using altmetrics to measure the impact of such dissemination.

SOCIAL MEDIA FOR CLINICAL PROFESSIONAL DEVELOPMENT

The pace of new knowledge in psychiatry continues to accelerate, and it is a challenge for any practicing psychiatrist to stay current on the latest articles. One advantage of Twitter is that it can serve as an "annotated bibliography" of new articles posted by journals, colleagues, organizations, and mentees. In the experience of the authors, social media is particularly helpful to learn about important papers published in fields outside of psychiatry. For example, there is a very strong group of female physicians organized under the #WomenInMedicine hashtag who frequently disseminate articles about gender equity in medicine. See **Table 2** for a list of psychiatric professional organizations on Twitter that typically disseminate articles relevant to all psychiatrists such as the American Psychiatric Association or to subspecialties such as the American Academy of Child & Adolescent Psychiatry. New practice guidelines, ethical guidelines, policies, and regulatory updates are frequently tweeted out by these organizations, which help members in practice stay familiar with the cutting edge updates in their fields.

MEDIA, ADVOCACY, AND PUBLIC POLICY

Psychiatrists are often called by the media to comment on important issues related to mental health. Common examples include being called in response to terrorist attacks, school shootings, and natural disasters such as hurricanes, floods, and wild fires. At other times, psychiatrists are called on to comment on public health issues, such as the impact of digital media on youth and adults, bullying, gun control, sexual assault, and other issues in the news. Psychiatrists should consider "striking while the iron is hot," as an analysis of 176 million tweets from 2011 to 2014 suggests that there is less than a 48-hour window after a depression- or suicide-related event when the public shows heightened interest in mental health.[21] Naturally, social media is a powerful means of conveying opinions and directing the public to evidence-based resources. It is often useful to post a psychiatrist's news clip, or interview with an online publication, and use Twitter to suggest other reputable sources of mental health information.

Although Twitter may be used for response to events in the news, another important role for psychiatrists is to proactively educate the public about mental health and the prevention of mental illness, define mental disorders, and help improve understanding and decrease stigma. For example, the lifetime prevalence of a psychiatric disorder is 24%, and 50% begins before age 14 years and 75% begin by age 26 years.[22] Many of these disorders may be prevented or mitigated with early intervention. However, only a fraction of individuals seek mental health services. Some of this is due to lack of access to care; but other reasons are based on stigma.

Psychiatrists' professional obligation in public health as well as with individual patients and families is to provide the best education they can about mental health and illness. Many individuals will seek help by going to their browsers and may well find misinformation or frankly biased information about mental health. Psychiatrists' use of social media helps the public to not only learn about problems and the range of treatments but how to find local resources for themselves or family members.

A second obligation is the obligation to provide advocacy for social, economic, and systems of care that may enhance health. By posting articles in the press, videos, or their own material, psychiatrists may have a significant impact on leaders in health care systems, politicians, advocacy groups, as well as health care professionals in

Table 4		
Behavioral health media, advocacy, and public policy organizations		
Organization	**Twitter Handle**	**Followers**
Behavioral Health Advocacy & Media Organizations		
Mental Health America	@MentalHealthAm	289,000
American Foundation for Suicide Prevention	@afspnational	82,300
National Council for Behavioral Health	@NationalCouncil	32,800
Child Mind Institute	@ChildMindInst	28,600
National Alliance on Mental Illness (NAMI) Advocacy	@NAMIAdvocacy	2700
Clay Center for Young Healthy Minds	@MGHClayCenter	1815
Public Policy Organizations		
National Institute of Mental Health (NIMH)	@NIMHgov	1.15 Million
Centers for Disease Control & Prevention (CDC)	@CDCgov	1.13 Million
National Alliance on Mental Illness (NAMI) Communicate	@NAMICommunicate	129,000
Robert Wood Johnson Foundation (RWJF)	@RWJF	103,000
National Institute on Drug Abuse (NIDA)	@NIDAnews	45,500
Psychiatric News	@PsychiatricNews	3931

Note, this is a sample in each category and is not meant to be inclusive. Followers were assessed on December 15, 2018 and will likely change by date of publication.
Data from Twitter. Available at: https://twitter.com/. Accessed Dec 15, 2018.

other specialties. See **Table 4** for a list of behavioral health advocacy, media, policy, and public health organizations.

The guidelines for posting material, particularly controversial material, such as homicide prevention, are complex. Naturally, psychiatrists may post their own opinions or refer to their own blogs or research papers. However, if they are employed by an academic institution or teaching hospital, never forget that social media posts, even if the user's bio states that "tweets are my own," may be interpreted as the position of the employing institution. Although the swift pace of Twitter may create the illusion that a tweet has disappeared, there is a permanence to these posts that requires a keen sense of judgment in case they are viewed months or years later when context is less clear.[4,23] A survey of 1314 emergency medicine residents and faculty found that both encountered frequent high-risk-to-professionalism events related to social media use by providers such as intoxicated colleagues, inappropriate photographs, identifiable patient information, and inappropriate posts.[24] Hence, it is always important when psychiatrists use social media, or when they are interviewed by the press, that they inform their public affairs office and ensure that their comments are acceptable to their institution. In other words, psychiatrists and physicians should strive to maintain a professional image and be mindful of the "digital footprints" they leave online and their potential impact on patients and families.[25]

SUMMARY

The use of social media is becoming increasingly common with each generation and psychiatrists must be familiar with the benefits and risks of this platform in creating a professional brand. Twitter can be especially helpful to psychiatrists due to the high numbers of organizations, journals, and discussions related to mental health policy, practice, research, and education. Its use in academic settings may drive greater networking with peers who share similar research or educational interests and can serve as a platform to amplify mentoring of trainees and colleagues. The field of altmetrics is emerging to quantify the impact of scholarly articles beyond the scientific community and can be a tool to measure the broader dissemination of research. For busy clinicians, Twitter offers a personalized bibliography of new articles annotated by respected colleagues and journals. There is an opportunity to use social media for advocacy through media and policy as well as to enhance public health. Although there is a degree of career risk with the use of social media, this can be moderated by a rule of thumb we call the "3 Ps." If psychiatrists ask themselves if they are comfortable with their message being read by their patients, their partners, and their public relations office, then they can proceed with sending the next tweet.

REFERENCES

1. Peters ME, Uible E, Chisolm MS. A Twitter education: why psychiatrists should tweet. Curr Psychiatry Rep 2015;17(12):94.
2. Smith A, Anderson M. Social media use in 2018. Pew Research Center 2018. Available at: http://www.pewinternet.org/wp-content/uploads/sites/9/2018/02/PI_2018.03.01_Social-Media_FINAL.pdf. Accessed December 15, 2018.
3. Pillow MT, Hopson L, Bond M, et al. Social media guidelines and best practices: recommendations form the council of residency directors social media task force. West J Emerg Med 2014;15(1):26–30.
4. Gregory K, Singh SS. Anger in academic Twitter: sharing, caring and getting mad online. TripleC 2018;16(1):176–93. Available at: https://www.triple-c.at/index.php/tripleC/article/view/890/1102.

5. Yellowlees P, Nafiz N. The psychiatrist-patient relationship of the future: anytime, anywhere? Harv Rev Psychiatry 2010;18:96–102.

6. Zalpuri I, Liu HY, Stubbe D, et al. Social media and networking competencies for psychiatric education: skills, teaching methods, and implications. Acad Psychiatry 2018;42:808–17.

7. Logghe HJ, Selby LV, Boeck MA, et al. The academic tweet: Twitter as a tool to advance academic surgery. J Surg Res 2018;226:8–12.

8. Elmously A, Salemi A, Guy TS. The anatomy of a tweet: social media in surgical practice. Semin Thorac Cardiovasc Surg 2018;30:251–5.

9. Adilman R, Rajmohan Y, Brooks E, et al. Social media use among physicians and trainees: results of a national medical oncology physician survey. J Oncol Pract 2016;12(1):79–80, e52–60.

10. Pearson D, Bond MC, Kegg J, et al. Evaluation of social media use by emergency medicine residents and faculty. West J Emerg Med 2015;16(50):715–20.

11. Using Twitter. Twitter help center. Available at: https://help.twitter.com/en/using-twitter. Accessed April 21, 2019.

12. Forgie SE, Duff JP, Ross S. Twelve tips for using twitter as learning tool in medical education. Med Teach 2013;35(1):8–14.

13. Diug B, Kendal E, Ilic D. Evaluating the use of Twitter as a tool to increase engagement in medical education. Educ Health (Abingdon) 2016;29(3):223–30.

14. Ke Q, Ahn Y-Y, Sugimoto CR. A systematic identification and analysis of scientists on Twitter. PLoS ONE 2017;12(4). Available at: https://www-ncbi-nlm-nih-gov.library1.unmc.edu/pmc/articles/PMC5388341/pdf/pone.0175368.pdf.

15. Côté IM, Darling ES. Scientists on Twitter: Preaching to the choir or singing from the rooftops?. FACETS, 3, 2018. p. 682–94. Available at: https://www.facetsjournal.com/doi/10.1139/facets-2018-0002.

16. Maggio LA, Leroux TC, Meyer HS, et al. #MedEd: exploring the relationship between altmetrics and traditional measures of dissemination in health professions education. Perspect Med Educ 2018;7:239–47.

17. Maggio LA, Myer HS, Artino AR. Beyond citation rates: a real-time impact analysis of health professions education research using altmetrics. Acad Med 2017;92(10):1449–55.

18. Quintana DS, Doan NT. Twitter article mentions and citations: an exploratory analysis of publications in the American Journal of Psychiatry. Am J Psychiatry 2016;173(2):194.

19. Chisolm MS. Altmetrics for medical educators. Acad Psychiatry 2017;41(4):460–6.

20. Knowlton SE, Paganoni S, Niehaus W, et al. Measuring the impact of research using conventional and alternative metrics. Am J Phys Med Rehabil 2019;98:331–8.

21. McClellan C, Ali MM, Mutter R, et al. Using social media to monitor mental health discussions – evidence from Twitter. J Am Med Inform Assoc 2017;24(3):496–502.

22. Kessler RC, Chiu WT, Demler O, et al. Prevalence, severity and comorbidity of 12-month DSM-IV disorders in the National Comorbidity Survey Replication. Arch Gen Psychiatry 2005;62(6):612–27.

23. Kind T. Professional guidelines for social media use: a starting point. AMA J Ethics 2015;17(5):441–7.

24. Garg M, Pearson DA, Bond MC, et al. Survey of individual and institutional risk associated with the use of social media. West J Emerg Med 2016;17(3):344–9.

25. Greysen SR, Kind T, Chretien KC. Online professionalism and the mirror of social media. J Gen Intern Med 2010;25(11):1227–9.

Role of Technology in Faculty Development in Psychiatry

Donald M. Hilty, MD, MBA[a],*, Jessica Uno, MD[b],
Steven Chan, MD, MBA[c], John Torous, MD[d], Robert J. Boland, MD[e]

KEYWORDS

- Technology • Education • Clinical • Development • Wellness • Career
- Lifelong learning • Social media

KEY POINTS

- Technology enhances clinical care, both in terms of daily practice options and strategies for providers and in terms of organizing, integrating, and evaluating practice systems.
- Pedagogic methods (ie, setting outcomes/expectations, teaching practices/interventions, and assessment/evaluation) previously supplemented by technology are now exponentially expanded by information technology innovations.
- Lifelong learning may occur via traditional (ie, book, in-person, scientific meeting) or contemporary digital options, which are easily accessible, affordable, and provide longitudinal integration.
- Faculty and career development is facilitated by technology, particularly in terms of professional identity, portfolios, provider and patient collaboration, networking, and practice management.
- Technology presents both challenges and benefits to work-life balance and integration.

INTRODUCTION

Clinicians, interprofessional teams, organization systems, and patients increasingly use technology for health and health care, as well as for communication, networking,

Disclosure Statement: The authors have nothing to disclose.
[a] Mental Health, Northern California Veterans Administration Health Care System, Department of Psychiatry and Behavioral Sciences, University of California Davis, 10535 Hospital Way, Mather, CA 95655, USA; [b] Psychiatry, Kaweah Delta Health Care District, 400 West Mineral King Avenue, Visalia, CA 93291, USA; [c] Addiction Treatment Services, Veterans Affairs Palo Alto Health Care System, University of California, San Francisco, 3801 Miranda Avenue, Building 520F, Mail Code 116A, Palo Alto, CA 94304, USA; [d] Digital Psychiatry Division, Department of Psychiatry, Beth Israel Deaconess Medical Center, 330 Brookline Avenue, Boston, MA 02115, USA; [e] Department of Psychiatry, Brigham and Women's Hospital, Harvard Medical School, 60 Fenwood Road, Boston, MA 02115, USA
* Corresponding author.
E-mail address: donh032612@gmail.com

Psychiatr Clin N Am 42 (2019) 493–512
https://doi.org/10.1016/j.psc.2019.05.013
0193-953X/19/© 2019 Elsevier Inc. All rights reserved.

psych.theclinics.com

and business. Psychiatric practice continues to evolve, as more care, education, and health resources are available online. Ubiquitous connectivity is now considered as vital as utilities such as water and electricity in both the educational and health care setting—hence, the period is described as the digital age.[1] Technology is also facilitating interprofessional collaboration, faculty and career development, and wellness in both professional and personal lives (**Fig. 1**).

Technology's reach extends beyond telepsychiatry/telebehavioral health via video-conferencing. Indeed, mobile health, apps, and smart devices provide new ways for patients and clinicians to connect—including children and adolescents—in ways that offer efficiency and are cost-effective.[2-5] Social media and networking, text messaging, e-mail, and other technologies are helping people stay fit and engage with others, while simultaneously presenting challenges to their focus and wellness when misused.[2,3,6] The impact of technology on the therapeutic relationship is key in 3 ways: in session, between sessions, and with technologies using simulation/virtual therapists.[2,6,7]

A paradigm shift has been in progress, moving from merely adding technologic options to existing processes, to using technology as essential, centralized tool for organization and facilitation. This may be conceptualized as a *shared information technology (IT)-business-medicine* understanding or model. This model improves performance via efficiency, managerial teamwork, quality of data, and data information processing and integration in business.[8] Successful companies ranging from L'Oreal to Cirque du Soleil and Nintendo have effectively integrated IT with research and development, marketing, production, and financing divisions.[9-11] Health care has seen similar corporatization, information revolution, globalization, and reform from its start as small businesses to large health care systems organized to serve the customer via patient-centered care models.[12]

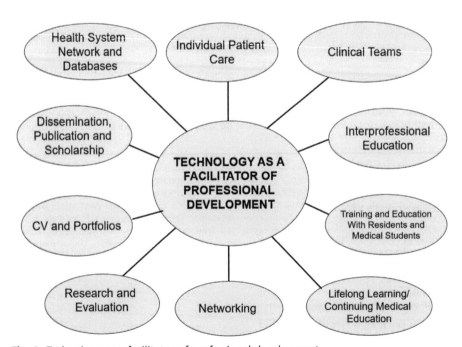

Fig. 1. Technology as a facilitator of professional development.

Lifelong learning (LLL) and faculty/career development are ongoing processes in clinical, research, and collaborative roles and attempt to balance professional/personal endeavors. The development of skills and attitude adjustment are pivotal—a regular feature of today's learning generation—and no longer "optional" for those in practice.[13,14] Measurable, desired outcomes for learners steer graduate and continuing medical education (CME; global medical education [GME]) and predetermine the learning setting, teaching methods used, and assessment and evaluation measures.[14] With regard to technology and clinical care, competencies are available for telepsychiatry in 2015, telebehavioral health in 2017, social media in 2018, and mobile health in 2019.[15–19] These help clinicians work with a broad range of technologies, known as an e-behavioral health spectrum, including Internet chat rooms, social media, online education, text messaging, mobile apps, and video production (**Table 1**).[2]

Day-to-day life is more facile on one hand, and more challenging, on the other, for everyone through technology. Technology alerts/prompts us nearly every hour of the day. Sometimes that is helpful and other times it may feel intrusive, particularly in a clinical therapy hour. Technology may interfere with basic cognitive processes that are associated with high(er) levels of happiness and lower levels of stress—specifically the contemplation of the future and weighing our prospects in making plans.[20] This is not surprising, because at least 3 facets of cognition are affected by these technologies—attention, memory, and reward processing (ie, delay of gratification). Thus, people including clinicians should be cautious about distractions from technologies, as we overestimate our ability to multitask.[3]

This article will help the reader consider ways to apply technology in his/her approach to the following:

1. Clinical care, by using it to add quality, efficiency, and evaluation, but prevent distractions and unnecessary labors;
2. LLL, teaching, and innovations through it;
3. Faculty and career development, as they develop their digital identity, develop their academic portfolio, manage a practice, and network and collaborate across distance; and
4. Wellness and balance with or integration of professional and personal obligations.

APPLYING TECHNOLOGY IN PROFESSIONAL WORK TO IMPROVE CLINICAL QUALITY, EFFICIENCY, AND EVALUATION

Psychiatric clinical practice and its governing evidence base continue to evolve and adapt to patient-centered care, which emphasizes quality, affordable, and timely health care.[21] Clinicians must learn a variety of models of care and systems (eg, value-based care [VBC] and accountable care organizations) that are driven by the Centers for Medicare and Medicaid Service (CMS) and the Affordable Care Act.[21] VBC has spurred the widespread deployment of technology in health care settings, most obviously electronic health records (EHRs) and telepsychiatry, because they facilitate access to care, leverages specialist consultation, and may reduce cost to the patient and clinicians. Areas include, but are not limited[22] to, the following:

Patient Care
- EHRs and clinical decision support
- Patient portals/open notes for psychiatry
- Electronic diagnostics and treatments
- Computer/mobile apps
- Telepsychiatry

Table 1
A continuum of technology use in health and clinical care: issues for patients and clinicians

Level	Source/Entry	Initiator Goals/Aims	Guiding Perspectives and Questions	Problems and Liabilities	Suggestions for Success
1	Website information	Person/patient: obtain health information and gain perspective. Clinician: provide valid, standard, and helpful info	Do I need more information? How should I approach the problem? What is out there? Better if referred by clinician who has checked it out	Quality of information and lack of regulation	Learn how to evaluate sites, information, and use it. Screen/have others for patients' use
2	Support/chat groups or communities	Person/patient: offers spontaneous, anonymous tips and perspective. Clinician: use to increase socialization and reduce isolation	Will this help and what should/can I do? What are others doing globally? Is the connection helpful or not for patients?	Peer compatibility? Information quality? Who is talking on the other end? How impressionable are the patients?	Discuss pros/cons of modality. Specific sites and groups specific to a purpose. Monitor over time
3	Social media/networking	Person/patient/caregiver: easy, convenient, and spontaneous. Clinician: rarely use; could/should screen if/what patients are doing, why, and impact. All: if purposeful and focused on one dimension, it could add to relationship	Can affect therapeutic alliance positively/negatively. Public information may be visible; it cannot be collected for analysis, though. Discuss, weigh pros/cons, address privacy, when to use/not use (eg, SI), and tracking (if any). Not billable care	Not HIPAA compliant? Undisclosed and/or impulsive use may indicate problems and boundary issues? Personal/professional role diffusion?	Provide skills, knowledge, and approaches in curriculum and with case conferences. Focus on developing professional role in transition from past personal experiences
4	Online formal educational materials	Person/patient: knowledge. Caregiver: education, support, and advice. Clinician: CME for knowledge and skills	Is this a good way to learn? I need "sound" info to make decisions for loved ones. CME implies good quality and peers' opinion may be helpful	No in-person learning/interaction. May not fit learning style. Knowledge is not skill	Obtain advice on good options. Evaluate quality. Provide good options linked to specific care stages

5	Self-directed assessment	Person/patient: tips to reflect, make changes, and get help. Caregiver: same and helped loved ones, too. Clinician: good for self- and life-long learning	What are my needs and resources? What is my next step in seeking help? Give patients assignments/ resources in conjunction with clinical care staff	Not all problems can be self-assessed and some illnesses affect insight and reflection	Evaluate options, take steps and share information with clinician. Support patients' and caregivers' initiative
6	Self-care decision-making options	Person/patient/caregiver: choose options and discuss impact with clinician. Clinician: empower patients and make assignments to needs	Can/should I make a change? Do I need more help? Who should I get advice from? Which of my patients can do some of this outside the office with help?	Should I do option A or B? How do I decide? Quality, context, and sequence is important	Evaluate options, take initiative, and discuss next/ new step with clinicians. Verify and provide good resources
7	Assisted self-care assessment and decision-making; deidentified	Person/patient/caregiver: feel ownership of care and better partnership. Clinician: distributes my time with help from others and empowers patients	Empowering and increased self-efficacy. Do I have time to discuss issues with patient or can my staff do that	Bad outcomes may occur with misstep or regular course. Doing too much without oversight is a risk?	Provide training on options, evaluating steps, and how to share information. Make decisions together
8	Asynchronous, between-session patient-clinician contact (eg, mobile app or e-mail/text)	Person/patient/caregiver: answer minor question, get a reminder. Clinician: good for quick advice and simple tasks (eg, assess mood, medication adherence)	Convenient to reach the clinician or team member? Easier for teen patients, who prefer texting over calling? Build into the EHR? Is the contact tracked, private, documented, and billable?	Some patients and/or clinicians do not use? Things taken out of context; errors? HIPAA compliant? Extra time to do	Help patients evaluate options, learn process. Simplify and directly link to care issue. Training on e-mail/text options and systems
9	Continuous mobile health/ e-monitoring to database/EHR	Person/patient/caregiver: as access to clinical team. Clinician: longitudinal monitoring, frequent contacts	Patient feels glad to be tracked, part of treatment, and "connected" to clinician. Integrated decision-making takes preparation and time?	Best in systematic care models with team-based approach?	All: set expectations and boundaries. Communication is key. Training, coordination, and documentation
10	Synchronous, traditional, or telebehavioral health care	Person/patient: it works and is much more convenient. Clinician: if patients like it, it is a good option	Allows synchronous decision-making (patient-clinician). Enhances links between clinicians and teams	It always has to be scheduled (and paid for); not spontaneous	Educate on pros/cons. Explore clinic- vs home-based models

Abbreviations: EHR, electronic health record; HIPAA, health insurance portability and accountability act.
Adapted from Hilty D, Chan S, Torous J, et al. New frontiers in healthcare and technology: internet-and web-based mental options emerge to complement in-person and telepsychiatric care options. J Health Med Informat 2015;6(4):200; with permission.

Communication
- Understanding patient use and barriers to technology
- In-person versus e-mail, telephone, and text
- Security/encryption and privacy
- Privacy
- Social media

Practice Management
- Professionalism
- Web presence
- Cloud resources/tools

Metrics and measures for quality care are increasingly emphasized and overseen by the CMS, Joint Commission, and other agencies. CMS uses a payment system that determines reimbursement on both the provision of a service and demonstration of quality care and improved patient health outcomes.[23] Behavioral health measures include suicide risk assessment, depression screening, and provision of a follow-up plan for positive screens. To minimize the survey and data burden for patients and clinicians, respectively, a reasonable approach may be to choose a widely used standard outcome measure and to anticipate regulatory and payer metrics (eg, Joint Commission's Standard CTS.03.01.09—for measurement-based care).[24] Overarching goals are to prioritize technologies implemented and to integrate technology into the overall workflow, which may include adjustments of consent, intake, and other administrative processes.

There are many technologies available, including mobile apps, audio-assisted EHRs, online scheduling (eg, Amion), and many others informed by artificial intelligence. Mobile apps and wearable devices have yet to be adopted widely in standard clinical practice, but the functionality is available. The benefit to mobile apps is their ease and widespread accessibility wherever the patient is located, relatively higher adoption than patient portals amongst lower-aged cohorts and patients of lower socioeconomic status.[25] The best approach is to use an evidence-based app in an evidence-based clinical intervention.[22,23] Apps that potentially enhance patient compliance, convenience, and access to care may still require more research and are not without risks of their own.[26] The American Psychiatric Association (APA) now recommends that psychiatrists follow an established protocol for evaluating the applications about which patients inquire.[27] Wearable devices such as the FitBit or Apple Watch can capture sleep patterns, activity level, and vital statistics such as heart rate or temperature. Patients can synchronize these to their own personal health record; in some cases, data can be entered into the EHR.

Technology poses some challenges to clinical practice and it is suggested to keep up-to-date, confer with others, and "step back" to see what daily operations may need adjustment.[22] As inferred earlier, technology distractions and suboptimal multitasking may affect attention, patient engagement, and the therapeutic alliance. Rapid and brief communications via text may lead to misunderstandings. Also, fatigue may be part of regular or overuse of technology, as increased access forces us (and trainees and patients) to try to figure out what is relevant and what is less relevant. Therefore, overall effectiveness, practicality,[28,29] and information curating[30] arise as themes. Cyberbullying and digital self-harm are being assessed by organizations such as the American Academy of Pediatrics and the American Academy of Child and Adolescent Psychiatry.[31–33] Mainstream news reports also debate about invalidated phenomenon such as "Snapchat dysmorphia" and "social media anxiety disorder."[33,34]

The field is moving more virtual in terms of clinical care but also for understanding how in-person, telepsychiatric, and other technologies affect communication, engagement, and the therapeutic relationship.[30] Indeed, virtual reality and its impact on users feeling present (ie, telepresence) is being researched across fields such as social neuroscience, neuroscience, the military (eg, Army), communication, computer science, tourism, robotics, artificial intelligence, virtual clinical interviewing, and mental health care.[35] The integration of communication technologies into supervisory practice also depends on presence, which enables supervisor and supervisee relationships to be in-person, online, or both. This model for future supervisory practice will be a "hybrid" relationship, similar to the patient-clinician relationship in-person and through technology. The major advantages over a purely in-person educational experience are convenience, extended reach to those in need, and overcoming cultural and/or language barriers.

LIFELONG LEARNING, TEACHING, AND INNOVATIONS THROUGH TECHNOLOGY

Traditionally, technology has not been considered, in and of itself, an educational method, but that is changing.[2,22] It has been seen rather as an alternative vehicle for delivering educational methods. In that regard, it has the advantage of often being able to deliver educational interviews more efficiently.[36] At the most basic level, online technologies deliver educational content as an analog and/or complement to traditional methods of pedagogy.[37] In addition, technologies can be used to explore more innovative approaches that harness the unique abilities of digital technology.

A broader perspective on the role of technology in education, and in clinical care, research, and other walks of life, may be realized by integrating practices of the US Department of Education's Office of Educational Technology Plan and Supplement[1] and business (eg, IBM[38]) with learning theory.[39] The perspective suggests that technology may affirm, accentuate, and augment our work. It may also complement existing practices, adding to, that is. Going further, it may help people explore, engage, and experiment with ideas and involved partners in new ways. In that sense, it "changes" dynamics or facilitates a different culture, which makes new things possible. Still further, technology may advance, engineer, and create completely new material—to truly innovate ideas and practices—in ways that were previously just not conceivable. This may be summarized as an *augmentation-exploration-innovation spectrum*.

Lecture-based learning is the most common, albeit least innovative form, of online teaching, with a recorded lecture delivered over the Internet instead of in-person. An advantage of this method is that it allows for asynchronous teaching and learning, at one's convenience. In addition, it allows for greater dissemination, as the lecture is not limited by room size or distance. Simply recording a live lecture for later online delivery may ignore some of the unique challenges of delivering online content. Remote or recorded lectures lack the feedback inherent during the classroom interaction and learners watching lectures remotely may not do so in a controlled environment (ie, without distraction).

As a result, some studies comparing video and live lectures suggest that there is better learning when there is a live interaction.[40] However, this clearly depends on the factors mentioned, and meta-analyses of existing studies do not support the superiority of live lectures; in fact there seems to be trend in favor of online lectures,[41] although there are several methodological limitations in these studies. The same studies, however, also suggest that the most effective teaching strategies are those that use combinations of the 2 or "blended learning."[42]

From a practical standpoint, those with cumulative experience in creating online lectures recommend several adaptations of the live presentation, including breaking down lectures into smaller chunks, preferably under 10 minutes, avoiding too much text on slides, and establishing a clear organization of content.[43] *Podcasts* are a good audio-only option and they differ from the above-described online lectures in style, delivery, and listener process (eg, mobile or on-the-go learner); many aspects, although, are similar to recorded live presentation.[44] Podcasts were originally designed for the listener who is doing other things such as driving, jogging, and cooking and who are now well-known in the business, journalist (ie, regular and investigative interviews), and medical fields. "Information on the go" is popular, as it delivers pieces of learning in small chunks. Typically, the style is less pedantic and favors a more informal, personal, and conversational approach to one-on-one engagement. These differences result in enjoyable and convenient ways to obtain CME credits, some of which are accompanied by online quizzes (see later discussion on board and practice-based learning changes).

Skill-based learning is a hallmark of medical education rather than just learning via lectures. Students practice skills in clinical situations under the supervision of a teacher who can then provide feedback and role model to shape the desired behaviors. Although a time-honored tradition in education, it is limited by the variability of experiences; ideally a student should encounter a great variety of situations and diagnoses, but these may not always be available during a time-limited clerkship. In addition, learning is optimized when students are allowed to explore situations, make mistakes, and learn from them; however, this has obvious ethical implications when practiced on actual patients. Technological strategies can address these limitations through the use of simulations. Simulations are increasingly used in medical settings, and studies suggest that high-fidelity simulations are both feasible and effective learning approaches.[45] Although often thought of as tools to teach procedural skills, they have also been used to teach more abstract concepts, such as team dynamics.[46]

Team-based learning is becoming a core practice in medical education, and, similar to problem-based learning, the classroom is "flipped" and the learners must work together to solve a problem or accomplish a goal with the teacher as a facilitator. Although most of the research investigating the efficacy of team-based learning has been done in live group settings, several educational institutions have adapted this approach to the online world, in which students must interact online and as a group must complete a project. Advantages of an online approach include the ability for asynchronous learning (ie, students log in and contribute at their convenience) and the ability of the approach to transcend distances and many sites. Several small studies have shown preliminary evidence to suggest that online team-based learning is feasible and effective.[47,48]

One challenge is keeping up to date on the evidence base, guidelines, and other resources. There are many ways to do this and most clinicians use a few new technologies in daily work (**Table 2**):

- Regular journal reading, grand rounds, practice group meetings, and case review
- Search engines connected with large databases (eg, PubMed) to carefully select new developments on a topic
- Membership in an organization (eg, ATA, APA): there are special conferences, extensive materials online (eg, APA Toolkit for telepsychiatry), list serves, and special interest groups
- Attending meetings with a technology focus (eg, ATA, APA, American Association for Technology in Psychiatry)

Table 2
Using technology for daily professional and personal development

Component	Description/Outcomes	Concerns/Bad Signs	Modern/Technology-Based Options to Help
Health and wellness			
Cognitive	Acquire knowledge via senses Facilitate attention and creativity	Forgetting context or key memories	Reminders, alarms, scheduling, and other structural/process options
Social	Meaningfully interact with others and be present even across distance	Isolation; disconnection via text content and/or symbols; withdrawal	Regular check-ins with friends, family, and peers
Physical	Build, organize program for energy	Fatigue	Health app, Fitbit-like device and other options
Emotional	Facilitate interest, passion, and coping; express empathy	Depression	Digital visual analog scale, mood rating, or emoticon estimation
Self-directed learning			
Case-based reading	Self-efficacy and knowledge on challenging issue	Superficial and/or too in-depth passages	Journals offer case series and CME
Individual journal clubs, webinars	Knowledge and resources on a new issue or recap of one	Multitasking	American Psychiatric Association and subspecialty organizations
Peer consultation: individual and/or group	Seek advice/perspective; gain shared understanding	Isolation; rote fixes that do not work	E-mail (if deidentified or private), telephone advice
CME in-depth course to target area	Knowledge, tips, and best practices on interests	Cost, time, and failure to apply to cases	Online courses readily available, including on required topics
Longitudinal series on a topic	Incremental learning with others	Inadequate time to prioritize	May require time and money but investment is good
Self- and peer assessment/reflection			
Assessment of errors or things we could do differently	Set aside time to review key decisions, weigh outcomes, and take preventive steps Diary for logging path and can search key terms	Bad outcomes with patients: medication errors, worsening delirium in an inpatient and/or suicide in an outpatient	EHR alerts, implementation of measurement-based care, prioritize digital questionnaires
Feedback from patients, peers, and systems	Ask patients periodically to inform care decisions Use meetings, conferences for support	Discontinuities in therapeutic relationship with patient or therapy not progressing	Improvement in Medical Practice (PIP) from American Board of Psychiatry and Neurology

(continued on next page)

			Modern/Technology-
Component	Description/Outcomes	Concerns/Bad Signs	Based Options to Help
Examination on clinical practice	Objective verification of knowledge and skills	Low scores, in general, and particularly in areas of interest	PIP Examination (PIPE) from American Board of Psychiatry and Neurology
Data-based feedback	Automated systems provide input on outcomes and decisions for planning	Perception of knowledge, skills, and other dimensions is (only) partially correct	EHR, personal health monitor for patient

Table 2
(continued)

- Journal membership (eg, Telemedicine and e-Health, Journal of Technology in Behavioral Sciences, Journal of Medical Informatics Mental Health)
- Online training (eg, Focus has modules consistent with the American Board of Psychiatry and Neurology's [ABPN] certification process)

In the future, there may be more online training, simulation, and/or interactive electronic examinations for psychiatry boards, using a culture of weekly to monthly learning rather than a quasi-annual or 10-year cycles of recertification based on examinations.[49,50] This dovetails with Part IV of ABPN, which is Improvement in Medical Practice (PIP), in which diplomates identify and implement areas for improvement based on review of their own patient charts (clinical module) or collect feedback on clinical performance from peers or patients via a questionnaire/survey (feedback module). This quality improvement exercise is designed for clinically active physicians to identify and implement areas for improvement within one's own practice.

Some professions are beginning to move from training and follow-up examination "steps" to a longitudinal series of "microsteps." The American College of Cardiology has rolled out the Lifelong Learning Portfolio, largely conducted via technology, and tools such as CardioCompass to search guidelines.[51] The Maintenance of Certification for Anesthesiology uses the MOCA Minute, an interactive learning tool being piloted to replace the Cognitive Examination. It consists of multiple-choice questions as those seen typically in MOC-Anesthesiology examinations—30 questions per calendar quarter.[49] Other examples include current practice podcasts accompanied by CME quizzes from the American Academy of Neurology (http://tools.aan.com/elibrary/continuum/index.cfm?event=podcast.selectexam); the American Journal of Psychiatry (https://ajp.psychiatryonline.org/audio); and the APA's own podcast list, which focus on current events and recent discoveries.[52]

FACULTY/CAREER DEVELOPMENT RELATED TO DIGITAL IDENTITY/ACADEMIC PORTFOLIO, MANAGE A PRACTICE AND NETWORK/COLLABORATE ACROSS DISTANCE

There are many faculty development implications for departments and academic health centers (AHCs) related to technology. At a minimum, departments, AHCs, and other provider organizations should create a set of social media policies and an annual training mechanism to update clinicians on the common risks of unprofessional behavior and privacy violations. This opportunity for real-time patient education and interaction reflects a larger trend termed "patient engagement," which is gaining traction in health care leadership.[53] Rather than having patients navigate impersonal

Websites, accurate health information can be posted by individual faculty members, departments of psychiatry, and AHCs via blogs, tweets, chats, and others. An effective patient engagement campaign requires a coordinated effort by public relations staff and departmental educators to review social media competencies, assess individual faculty member's expertise levels via interactive workshops, and model best practices with the help of social media innovators and experts.

Developing an academic portfolio is also facilitated technology, with materials being best practices and standardization. For example, a national training library of interactive social media vignettes would allow standardization of clinical and professional development training across institutions. This technique has been demonstrated by the Association of Directors of Medical Student Education in Psychiatry Clinical Simulation Initiative—a free online peer-reviewed compilation of psychiatric cases for medical student education—accessed more than 73,919 times between 2013 and 2017.[54]

Practice management includes a wide range of activities, including clinical, marketing, administrative, and regulatory aspects. Management technology is already well-integrated into such processes as organizing providers' appointment schedules, verifying patient insurance information, and managing billing cycles). More recently, IT in the form of social media is gaining a prominent position in practice management and professional development. Social media is defined as web-based tools or "applications" that generally facilitate direct-to-consumer delivery of media and information.[55] It emphasizes both connections between individuals and "broadcasting" of messages and ideas from one source to many. In considering the clinician's approach to social media, it may be useful to conceptualize the utility of social media into 3 domains: content intended for

1. A professional audience,
2. A patient audience, and
3. A combination public audience (**Fig. 2**).

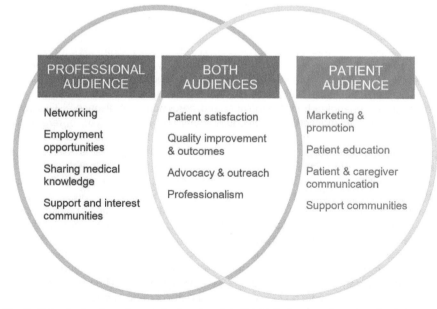

Fig. 2. Using technology for professional and patient relations and communication.

Many social media apps can be used in more than one domain.

Social media is key in building and projecting an identity with which both professional and patient audiences can connect. There are a variety of options available online for projecting one's professional persona. Multimedia platforms such as blogs, vlogs, and podcasts are common, as are social media options such as Facebook and Twitter.[20] This digital identity, more commonly known as a "profile,"can be disseminated for the purposes of professional networking (exemplified by communities such as LinkedIn and Doximity), showcasing one's work (via online portfolios), and position recruitment and job opportunities. The social media platforms for projecting one's professional identity include both general (ie, LinkedIn) and health care profession-specific varieties (Doximity). Among colleagues and peers, social media can promote positive connectivity that decrease feelings of isolation and strengthens professional communities via forum and messaging applications.[56]

Media also facilitates engagement with patient audiences, encompassing direct patient-provider communication and patient education, as well as encouraging patient referrals via friends and family. Research shows that effective self-promotion, patient education, sharing of medical knowledge, and patient satisfaction/quality assessments can be accomplished via social media.[57] A particular example of rising attention are "crowdsourced" hospital/provider ratings, which compile direct consumer feedback about individual providers into simplified "grades" that are shared with the public. Examples of online avenues for patient satisfaction assessments include HealthGrades, Google Business, and Yelp. Oftentimes, the profiles on these sites are not created by the provider themselves but they are drawn from public record and provide a sounding board for both pleased and dissatisfied patients to share their experiences. Providers have limited ability to edit or curate the content added by consumers on their profiles. Studies show conflicting evidence for how accurately or precisely these consumer-centric, crowdsourced ratings capture the performance of a provider.[58,59] Currently, there is limited utility and relevance of patient feedback from review Websites, and the impact they should have on real-world practice is still up for debate.[60] Some suggest that when executed in a rigorous and evidence-driven manner however, crowdsourcing could potentially become a powerful tool for research.[61]

Social media in medical professional identity has notably been used to promote awareness and education among professionals and laypersons for various disease-specific causes. This phenomenon is known as the "social media campaign," and it has been widely and successfully used to garner financial, social, and political support directed toward changing health behaviors and perceptions of disease.[62] This strategy has successfully highlighted traditionally lesser known, neglected, or rare health conditions, especially when paired with "crowdfunding campaigns" that encourage large-scale grassroot donations to health causes.[63] One example is the #BPDCN Twitter campaign that focused on a rare malignancy and ultimately promoted increased scientific discussion, researcher engagement, and caregiver/patient supportgroups.[64] In psychiatry alone, significant attention has been directed toward mental health issues, thanks to recent "social media campaigns" following highly publicized tragedies.[65] Looking forward, social media may be a viable platform for driving research funding and intervention implementation.

Social media is a pervasive platform for support communities, academic discussions, and the direct dissemination of new knowledge quickly and cheaply. As fluid as social media identity is, however, steps must always be taken in any of the above-mentioned domains to avoid privacy violations and the blurring of boundaries between personal and professional lives and image.[57]

BOOSTING WELLNESS AND BALANCING LIFE'S ROLES VIA TECHNOLOGY

Technology's practicality promises improvements toward the Triple Aim of patient experience of care, the health of populations, and the cost of health care.[66] Technology can address a fourth aim to address widespread burnout and dissatisfaction amongst health care providers by improving the work life of such providers and staff.[67]

There is an increased focus on physician burnout, physician suicide,[68] and wellness.[69] Physicians work best when they take care of themselves and feel supported.[70–72] Wellness is essential to maintain high-quality patient care, as physicians are providers and leaders within the health system. About 15% of physicians during their professional lifetimes will develop a substance abuse– and/or mental health–related condition, which may potentially impair their ability to practice medicine to the best of their ability.[73,74] Related concerns are those of physician burnout, depression, neurocognitive impairment, disruptive behavior, and suicide.[75–77] Professional wellness is not just altruistic care for colleagues but also benefits patients, because professionals work best when they care for themselves.[77]

To prevent burnout, *self-care* can help providers set boundaries. However, no single definition of self-care is broadly accepted in the literature, as definitions vary as to who engages in self-care behavior, what motivates self-care behavior, and the extent to which health care professionals are involved.[78] Likewise, the concepts of wellness, happiness, joy, stress, and coping are applied to self-care. A simple definition of wellness is a good or satisfactory condition of existence; a state characterized by health, happiness, and prosperity.[79] From a different perspective, the absence of control or the loss of real or perceived control can cause problems, whereas those with an internal locus of control feel empowered to cope with stress.

A variety of web-based or mobile tools applied to improve patient care may also be applied to clinician self-care. For instance, in a randomized controlled trial of 199 hospital interns across multiple specialties, web-based CBT application MoodGYM was found to reduce suicidal ideation as reported by the PHQ-9.[80] Five particular categories of web-based and mobile applications have been identified as having effectiveness for health care students and providers in the areas of cognitive behavioral therapy, meditation, mindfulness, breathing, and relaxation techniques, and a recent *Academic Psychiatry* paper enumerates 36 distinct resources.[81]

Coping with professional and personal matters, changes, and other events requires emotional, physical, and social resources (see **Table 2**). Coping is an effortful process that requires resources such as health and energy, positive belief, problem-solving skills, social skills, social support, and material. Self-reflection and meditation at the start/end of the day, a quick walk midday to clear the confusion and stress, and asking for ideas rather than telling others what to do helps. Healthy and robust individuals are better able to cope, so regular exercise keeps us in shape and may inoculate us to repeated exposure to moderate levels of physical stress. Another important factor in health is sleep, which many learn in medical school or from having children to be a luxury rather than a necessity.

Many specific practices of self-care and coping come from the world of business and entertainment (eg, games), but research in neuroscience reveals the common issues.[82] For instance, limiting use of digital devices after hours—for instance, placing devices in specific containers and setting boundaries around use—can prevent the intrusion of work into personal life and periods of self-care. Deliberate scheduling of restorative, downtime activities during the workday, weekends, and off-hours can reduce stress.[83]

Improving specific work technologies can reduce stress and burnout. Clinical informatics consensus is that the EHR, when poorly designed, can frustrate providers, lead to burnout, and cause increased staff turnover. Technologies such as EHRs and always-connected smartphones have given clinicians the ability to work anywhere and anytime. This flexibility has led to clinicians to take homework at night, writing notes, reviewing messages, and prescribing remotely to essentially complete clerical tasks.[84] Improving the efficiency of the EHR,[85] along with greater empowerment and resources over their workflow and environment in parallel with Len Schlesinger's service profit chain framework,[86] can alleviate burnout. Because many current EHRs have decades-old user interfaces that requires clicks, software developers can use voice-driven user interfaces, data visualizations, and artificial intelligence augmentation to boost the usability of these interfaces and help cut through duplicative documentation requirements and demands.[87] Both patient workloads and stress caused by EHR should be measured.[88]

Finally, *social skills and support*, including those accessed via technology, refer to a broad repertoire of behaviors that allow one to interact with others in a meaningful and respectful manner. Social support includes 4 primary factors:

1. Emotional concern (expressing empathy and caring),
2. Instrumental aid (giving and receiving assistance),
3. Information (giving and receiving advice, directions, and suggestions), and
4. Appraisal (feedback from the other person's appraisal).[89]

The rise of telemental health services providing video psychotherapy helps technology address provider privacy concerns, scheduling conflicts, and travel time barriers[90,91] but further improvement needs to help address provider licensing, prescription ordering, and insurance reimbursement barriers.[92]

SUMMARY

New developments in psychiatry, medicine, and science, coupled with changes in health care and practice, make it imperative that clinicians adapt to and adopt technology and help patients to do the same to ensure quality, affordable, and timely care. Service delivery more and more includes technology, in the form of EHR, communication (eg, text, e-mail, social media), and care modalities (eg, telepsychiatry). Technology application and integration to workflow is essential. Building and maintaining skills – regardless of the degree of experience with clinical care and technology – requires clinicians to balance reasonable expectations and excitement about innovation. Purposeful use, ongoing discussion, and joint decision-making between clinicians and patients are needed to implement and evaluate such interventions, while weighing the pros and cons of technologies.

The digital age has solidified the role of technology in LLL, faculty/career development, and CME. Indeed, a paradigm shift has been in progress, moving from adding technology options to what we do, to using it as a central, organizing, and facilitating tool. This may be conceptualized as a *shared IT-business-medicine* understanding or model. Other fields of medicine are also adapting to the digital age, as are GME, undergraduate medical education, and other professional organizations in mental health, behavioral science, social sciences, and cultural anthropology. Online training, with simulated and/or electronic patients, a focus on skill development, team-based care, and communication will become commonplace. As with recent changes in GME accreditation, perhaps CME and board certification will shift from cross-sectional examinations over 10-year cycles to a monthly model of participation. Some specialties are already well underway.

Maintaining wellness is a foundation for making good care possible, as the psychiatrist is faced with balancing clinical care, teaching/education, research/evaluation, administration, and other roles. More research is needed on how technology helps and hinders. Indeed, the potential broader perspective that technology has much more impact—perhaps on an *augmentation-exploration-innovation* spectrum—also deserves greater consideration.

ACKNOWLEDGMENTS

The authors wish to acknowledge the following organizations: American Psychiatric Association and Telepsychiatry Committee, American Telemedicine Association and Telemental Health Interest Group, *Journal of Technology in Behavioral Science*, Springer–Nature Publishing.

REFERENCES

1. Office of Educational Technology. Reimagining the role of technology in education: 2017 national education technology plan update. 2017. Available at: https://tech.ed.gov/files/2017/01/NETP17.pdf. Accessed April 24, 2019.
2. Hilty DM, Chan S, Torous J, et al. New frontiers in healthcare and technology: Internet- and web-based mental options emerge to complement in-person and telepsychiatric care options. J Health Med Inform 2015;6(4):1–14.
3. Hilty DM, Chan S. Human behavior with mobile health: smartphone/devices, apps and cognition. Psychol Cogn Sci 2018;4(2):36–47.
4. Archangeli C, Marti FA, Wobga-Pasiah EA, et al. Mobile health interventions for psychiatric conditions in children: a scoping review. Child Adolesc Psychiatr Clin N Am 2017;26(1):13–31.
5. Powell AC, Chen M, Thammachart C. The economic benefits of mobile apps for mental health and telepsychiatry services when used by adolescents. Child Adolesc Psychiatr Clin N Am 2017;26(1):125–33.
6. Schueller SM, Stiles-Shields C, Yarosh L. Online treatment and virtual therapists in child and adolescent psychiatry. Child Adolesc Psychiatr Clin N Am 2017; 26(1):1–12.
7. Krishna R. The impact of health information technology on the doctor-patient relationship in child and adolescent psychiatry. Child Adolesc Psychiatr Clin N Am 2017;26(1):67–75.
8. Ray G, Muhanna WA, Barney JB. Competing with IT: the role of shared IT-business understanding. CommunACM 2007;50(12):87–91.
9. Emerald Group Publishing Group. Survival through innovation: microsoft and nintendo strive to offer the latest "must haves". Strategic Direction 2007;24(1):21–4. Available at: https://doi.org/10.1108/02580540810839313. Accessed June 15, 2019.
10. Rivard S, Pinsonneault A. Information technology at Cirque du Soleil: looking back, moving forward. Int J Case Stud Manag 2012;10(4):1–13. Available at: https://hbr.org/product/information-technology-at-cirque-du-soleil-looking-back-moving-forward/HEC039-PDF-ENG. Accessed June 15, 2019.
11. Dubois DBK. Ombre, tie-dye, splat hair: trends or fads?. In: "Pull" and "push" social media strategies at L'Oreal Paris. Insead; 2014.
12. Committee on Quality of Health Care in America, Institute of Medicine. Crossing the quality chasm: a new health system for the 21st century. National Academies Press; 2001.

13. Iobst WF, Sherbino J, Cate OT, et al. Competency-based medical education in postgraduate medical education. Med Teach 2010;32(8):651–6.
14. Snell LS, Frank JR. Competencies, the tea bag model, and the end of time. Med Teach 2010;32(8):629–30.
15. Hilty DM, Crawford A, Teshima J, et al. A framework for telepsychiatric training and e-health: Competency-based education, evaluation and implications. Int Rev Psychiatry 2015;27(6):569–92.
16. Hilty DM, Maheu M, Drude K, et al. The need to implement and evaluate telehealth. Acad Psychiatry 2018;42(6):818–24.
17. Maheu MM, Drude KP, Hertlein KM, et al. An interprofessional framework for telebehavioral health competencies. J Technol Behav Sci 2017;2(3–4):190–210.
18. Hilty DM, Zalpuri I, Stubbe D, et al. Social media/networking and psychiatric education: competencies, teaching methods, and implications. J Technol Behav Sci 2018;19:722.
19. Hilty DM, Chan S, Torous J, et al. A telehealth framework for mobile health, smartphones and apps: competencies, training and faculty development. J Technol Behav Sci 2019. https://doi.org/10.1007/s41347-019-00091-0 or. Available at: http://link.springer.com/article/10.1007/s41347-019-00091-0.
20. Seligman MEP, Tierney J. We aren't built to live in the moment. NY Times 2017.
21. Shi L, Singh DA. Delivering health care in America. 6th edition. Burlington (MA): Jones & Bartlett Learning; 2014.
22. Hilty DM, Turvey C, Hwang T. Lifelong learning for clinical practice: how to leverage technology for telebehavioral health care and digital continuing medical education. Curr Psychiatry Rep 2018;20(3):15.
23. National Direct Service Workforce Resource Center. Coverage of direct service workforce continuing education and training within Medicaid policy and rate setting: a Toolkit for state Medicaid agencies. Centers for Medicare & Medicaid Services; 2013. p. 12. Available at: https://www.medicaid.gov/medicaid/ltss/downloads/workforce/dsw-training-rates-toolkit.pdf.
24. The Joint Commission. Measurement-based care in behavioral health. Presented at the: The Joint Commission: Webinars and Education; April 11, 2017; Online. Available at: https://www.jointcommission.org/assets/1/6/bhc_Joint_Commission_measures_webinar_041117.pdf. Accessed June 15, 2019.
25. Chan S, Godwin H, Gonzalez A, et al. Review of use and integration of mobile apps into psychiatric treatments. Curr Psychiatry Rep 2017;19(12):96.
26. Top 25 mental health apps for 2018: an alternative to therapy? PsyCom.net - mental health treatment resource since 1986. Available at: https://www.psycom.net/25-best-mental-health-apps. Accessed June 15, 2019.
27. Mental health apps. Available at: https://www.psychiatry.org/psychiatrists/practice/mental-health-apps. Accessed June 15, 2019.
28. Ancker JS, Edwards A, Nosal S, et al. Effects of workload, work complexity, and repeated alerts on alert fatigue in a clinical decision support system. BMC Med Inform Decis Mak 2017;17. https://doi.org/10.1186/s12911-017-0430-8.
29. Yamamoto Y. Healthcare and the roles of the medical profession in the big data era. Japan Med Assoc J 2016;59(2–3):125–39.
30. Azim A, et al. Editorial processes in free open access medical educational (FOAM) resources. Available at: https://www.ncbi.nlm.nih.gov/pubmed/30051090. Accessed June 15, 2019.
31. Sussman N, DeJong SM. Ethical considerations for mental health clinicians working with adolescents in the digital age. CurrPsychiatry Rep 2018;20(12):113.

32. Bully and cyberbullying. Available at: https://www.aap.org/en-us/advocacy-and-policy/aap-health-initiatives/resilience/Pages/Bullying-and-Cyberbullying.aspx. Accessed June 15, 2019.

33. AACAP.Social networking and children. Available at: https://www.aacap.org/AACAP/Families_and_Youth/Facts_for_Families/FFF-Guide/Children-and-Social-Networking-100.aspx. Accessed June 15, 2019.

34. Rajanala S, Maymone MBC, Vashi NA. Selfies—living in the era of filtered photographs. JAMA Facial Plast Surg 2018. https://doi.org/10.1001/jamafacial.2018.0486.

35. Hilty DM, Randhawa R, Maheu M, et al. Quality telepractice and the therapeutic relationship: learning from virtual reality, augmented reality and telepresence. PsycholCognSci 2019. Available at: https://openventio.org/wp-content/uploads/Therapeutic-Relationship-of-Telepsychiatry-and-Telebehavioral-Health-Ideas-from-Research-on-Telepresence-Virtual-Reality-and-Augmented-Reality-PCSOJ-5-145.pdf.

36. Verduin ML, Boland RJ, Guthrie TM. New directions in medical education related to psychiatry. Int Rev Psychiatry 2013;25(3):338–46.

37. Means B, Toyama Y, Murphy R, et al. Evaluation of evidence-based practices in online learning: a meta-analysis and review of online learning studies. U.S. Department of Education, Office of Planning, Evaluation, and Policy Development; 2009. Available at: http://files.eric.ed.gov/fulltext/ED505824.pdf. Accessed April 24, 2019.

38. Levy F, Murnane RJ. A role for technology in professional development?Lessons from IBM. Phi Delta Kappan 2004;85(10):728–34.

39. Matzen NJ, Edmunds JA. Technology as a catalyst for change. J Res Tech Educ 2007;39(4):417–30. Available at: https://eric.ed.gov/?id=EJ768887. Accessed June 15, 2019.

40. Varao-Sousa TL, Kingstone A. Memory for lectures: how lecture format impacts the learning experience. PLoS One 2015;10(11):e0141587.

41. Means B, Toyama Y, Murphy R, et al. The effectiveness of online and blended learning: a meta-analysis of the empirical literature. Teach Coll Rec 2013;115(3).

42. Munro V, Morello A, Oster C, et al. E-learning for self-management support: introducing blended learning for graduate students - a cohort study. BMC Med Educ 2018;18(1):219.

43. Moore EA. Adapting PowerPoint lectures for online delivery: best practices. Faculty focus | Higher Ed teaching & learning 2013. Available at: https://www.facultyfocus.com/articles/online-education/adapting-powerpoint-lectures-for-online-delivery-best-practices/. Accessed April 24, 2019.

44. Kapoor S, Catton R, Khalil H. An evaluation of medical student-led podcasts: what are the lessons learnt? Adv Med Educ Pract 2018;9:133.

45. Armenia S, Thangamathesvaran L, Caine AD, et al. The role of high-fidelity team-based simulation in acute care settings: a systematic review. Surg J (N Y) 2018;4(3):e136–51.

46. Patterson MD, Geis GL, Falcone RA, et al. In situ simulation: detection of safety threats and teamwork training in a high risk emergency department. BMJQualSaf 2013;22(6):468–77.

47. Wong G, Greenhalgh T, Pawson R. Internet-based medical education: a realist review of what works, for whom and in what circumstances. BMC Med Educ 2010;10:12.

48. Mash RJ, Marais D, Van Der Walt S, et al. Assessment of the quality of interaction in distance learning programmesutilising the Internet (WebCT) or interactive television (ITV). Med Educ 2005;39(11):1093–100.

49. Bjork RA. Commentary on the potential of the MOCAminute program®. Anesthesiology 2016;125(5):844–5.

50. Moran M. ABPN to pilot new test format for maintenance of certification in 2019. Psychiatr News 2017;52(24):1.

51. Zoghbi WA, Beliveau ME. President's page: lifelong learning in the digital age. J Am CollCardiol 2012;60(10):944–6.

52. Podcasts. Available at: https://www.psychiatry.org/psychiatrists/education/podcasts. Accessed April 24, 2019.

53. Markham MJ, Gentile D, Graham DL. Social media for networking, professional development, and patient engagement. Am Soc Clin Oncol Educ Book 2017; 37:782–7.

54. Hawa R, Klapheke M, Liu H, et al. An innovative technology blueprint for medical education: association of directors of medical student education in psychiatry's clinical simulation initiative years 1-6. Acad Psychiatry 2017;41(3):408–10.

55. Ventola CL. Social media and health care professionals: benefits, risks, and best practices. P T 2014;39(7):491–520.

56. Pimmer C, Brühlmann F, Odetola TD. Instant messaging and nursing students' clinical learning experience. Available at: https://www.ncbi.nlm.nih.gov/pubmed/29475195. Accessed April 24, 2019.

57. Alshakhs F, Alanzi T. The evolving role of social media in health-care delivery: measuring the perception of health-care professionals in Eastern Saudi Arabia. J Multidiscip Healthc 2018;11:473–9.

58. Perez V, Freedman S. Do crowdsourced hospital ratings coincide with hospital compare measures of clinical and nonclinical quality? HealthServ Res 2018. https://doi.org/10.1111/1475-6773.13026.

59. Greaves F. Associations between web-based patient ratings and objective measures of hospital quality. Arch Intern Med 2012;172(5):435.

60. Glover M, Khalilzadeh O, Choy G, et al. Hospital evaluations by social media: a comparative analysis of facebook ratings among performance outliers. J Gen Intern Med 2015;30(10):1440–6.

61. Armstrong AW, Cheeney S, Wu J, et al. Harnessing the power of crowds: crowdsourcing as a novel research method for evaluation of acne treatments. Am J ClinDermatol 2012;13(6):405–16.

62. Freeman B, Potente S, Rock V, et al. Social media campaigns that make a difference: what can public health learn from the corporate sector and other social change marketers? PublicHealth Res Pract 2015;25(2):e2521517.

63. Koole MA, Kauw D, Winter MM, et al. A successful crowdfunding project for eHealth research on grown-up congenital heart disease patients. Available at: https://www.ncbi.nlm.nih.gov/pubmed/30297187. Accessed April 24, 2019.

64. Pemmaraju N, Utengen A, Gupta V. Blasticplasmacytoid dendritic cell neoplasm (bpdcn) on social media: #bpdcn-increasing exposure over two years since inception of a disease-specif. Available at: https://www.ncbi.nlm.nih.gov/pubmed/30338458. Accessed April 24, 2019.

65. Keane L. 5 mental health campaigns that made a difference | GlobalWebIndex.-GlobalWebIndex Blog. 2017. Available at: https://blog.globalwebindex.com/marketing/mental-health/. Accessed April 24, 2019.

66. The IHItriple aim. Available at: http://www.ihi.org/Engage/Initiatives/TripleAim/Pages/default.aspx. Accessed April 24, 2019.

67. Bodenheimer T, Sinsky C. From triple to quadruple aim: care of the patient requires care of the provider. Ann Fam Med 2014;12(6):573–6.
68. Goldman ML, Shah RN, Bernstein CA. Depression and suicide among physician trainees: recommendations for a national response. JAMA Psychiatry 2015;72(5): 411–2.
69. Panagioti M, Geraghty K, Johnson J, et al. Association between physician burnout and patient safety, professionalism, and patient satisfaction: a systematic review and meta-analysis. JAMA Intern Med 2018;178(10):1317–30.
70. Thomas MR, Dyrbye LN, Huntington JL, et al. How do distress and well-being relate to medical student empathy? A multicenter study. J Gen Intern Med 2007;22(2):177–83.
71. West CP, Huschka MM, Novotny PJ, et al. Association of perceived medical errors with resident distress and empathy: a prospective longitudinal study. JAMA 2006;296(9):1071–8.
72. Schwartz C, Meisenhelder JB, Ma Y, et al. Altruistic social interest behaviors are associated with better mental health. Psychosom Med 2003;65(5):778–85.
73. Boisaubin EV, Levine RE. Identifying and assisting the impaired physician. Am J Med Sci 2001;322(1):31–6.
74. Baldisseri MR. Impaired healthcare professional. CritCare Med 2007;35(Suppl): S106–16.
75. Moutier C, Cornette M, Lehrmann J, et al. When residents need health care: stigma of the patient role. AcadPsychiatry 2009;33(6):431–41.
76. Stack S. Suicide risk among physicians: a multivariate analysis. Arch Suicide Res 2004;8(3):287–92.
77. Haskins J, Carson JG, Chang CH, et al. The suicide prevention, depression awareness, and clinical engagement program for faculty and residents at the University of California, Davis Health System. AcadPsychiatry 2016;40(1):23–9.
78. Godfrey CM, Harrison MB, Lysaght R, et al. Care of self - care by other - care of other: the meaning of self-care from research, practice, policy and industry perspectives. Int J EvidBasedHealthc 2011;9(1):3–24.
79. Corbett B, Marla V, Nanda N, et al. Managing your time. In: Roberts LW, Hilty DM, editors. Handbook of career development in academic psychiatry and behavioral sciences. 2nd edition. Washington, DC: American Psychiatric Pub; 2017.
80. Guille C, Zhao Z, Krystal J, et al. Web-based cognitive behavioral therapy intervention for the prevention of suicidal ideation in medical interns: a randomized clinical trial. JAMA Psychiatry 2015;72(12):1192–8.
81. Pospos S, Young IT, Downs N, et al. Web-based tools and mobile applications to mitigate burnout, depression, and suicidality among healthcare students and professionals: a systematic review. AcadPsychiatry 2018;42(1):109–20.
82. Wilmer HH, Sherman LE, Chein JM. Smartphones and cognition: a review of research exploring the links between mobile technology habits and cognitive functioning. Front Psychol 2017;8:605.
83. How to overcome burnout and stay motivated. Harvard business review. Available at: https://hbr.org/2015/04/how-to-overcome-burnout-and-stay-motivated. Accessed April 24, 2019.
84. Wright AA, Katz IT. Beyond burnout - redesigning care to restore meaning and sanity for physicians. N Engl J Med 2018;378(4):309–11.
85. One way to prevent clinician burnout. Harvard business review. Available at: https://hbr.org/2017/10/one-way-to-prevent-clinician-burnout. Accessed April 24, 2019.

86. Giving doctors what they need to avoid burnout. Harvard business review. Available at: https://hbr.org/2017/10/giving-doctors-what-they-need-to-avoid-burnout. Accessed April 24, 2019.

87. To combat physician burnout and improve care, fix the electronic health record. Harvard business review. Available at: https://hbr.org/2018/03/to-combat-physician-burnout-and-improve-care-fix-the-electronic-health-record. Accessed April 24, 2019.

88. Linzer M, Levine R, Meltzer D, et al. 10 bold steps to prevent burnout in general internal medicine. J Gen Intern Med 2014;29(1):18–20.

89. House JS. Barriers to work stress: I. Social support. In: Behavioral medicine: work, stress and health. Reading (MA): Springer; 1985. p. 157–80.

90. Palus S. The online therapy services we'd use. Wirecutter: reviews for the real world. 2018. Available at: https://thewirecutter.com/reviews/online-therapy-services/. Accessed April 24, 2019.

91. Palus S. What is it like to use online therapy? Wirecutter: reviews for the real world. Available at: https://thewirecutter.com/blog/online-therapy-experience/.

92. Morland LA, Poizner JM, Williams KE, et al. Home-based clinical video teleconferencing care: clinical considerations and future directions. Int Rev Psychiatry 2015;27(6):504–12.

Mobile Health, Smartphone/ Device, and Apps for Psychiatry and Medicine
Competencies, Training, and Faculty Development Issues

Donald M. Hilty, MD, MBA[a],*, Steven Chan, MD, MBA[b],
John Torous, MD[c], John Luo, MD[d], Robert J. Boland, MD[e]

KEYWORDS

- Apps • Training • Mobile • Smartphone • Competencies • Health • Medicine
- Psychiatry

KEY POINTS

- Technology use is ubiquitous in the digital age; to ensure quality care, faculty and trainees need clinical skills, knowledge, and attitudes.
- An approach is needed to implement, teach, supervise, and evaluate clinical mobile health, smartphone/device, and app competences.
- Milestone domains of patient care, medical knowledge, practice-based learning and improvement, systems-based practice, professionalism, and interpersonal skills and communication may be used to organize these competencies.
- Faculty, department, and institutional approaches are needed to integrate mobile health into service delivery.

Disclosure Statement: The authors have nothing to disclose.
[a] Mental Health, Northern California Veterans Administration Health Care System, Department of Psychiatry and Behavioral Sciences, University of California Davis, 10535 Hospital Way, Mather, CA 95655, USA; [b] Addiction Treatment Services, Veterans Affairs Palo Alto Health Care System, University of California, San Francisco, 3801 Miranda Avenue, Building 520F, Mail Code 116A, Palo Alto, CA 94304, USA; [c] Digital Psychiatry Division, Department of Psychiatry, Beth Israel Deaconess Medical Center, 330 Brookline Avenue, Boston, MA 02215, USA; [d] UC Riverside Department of Psychiatry, UCR Health at Citrus Tower, 3390 University Avenue, Suite 115, Riverside, CA 92501, USA; [e] Department of Psychiatry, Brigham and Women's Hospital, Harvard Medical School, 60 Fenwood Road, Boston, MA 02115, USA
* Corresponding author.
E-mail address: donh032612@gmail.com

Psychiatr Clin N Am 42 (2019) 513–534
https://doi.org/10.1016/j.psc.2019.05.007
0193-953X/19/© 2019 Elsevier Inc. All rights reserved.

INTRODUCTION

Mobile communications smartphones and other devices (SP/D) supported by 3G and 4G mobile networks for data transport, computing and integration have been a force in business, entertainment and health communities. Mobile health and social media are propelled by the X, millennial/Y, and Z generations, delivering health care anytime and anywhere, and surpassing geographic, cost, temporal, and even organizational barriers.[1] This movement is consistent with person- and patient-centered care—known as participatory medicine—which moves patients from being mere passengers to responsible drivers of their health and as valued partners by physicians (persons will be called people going forward).[2] Accordingly, educational reform with technology is suggested by the World Health Organization[3] and the Institute of Medicine.[4,5]

In health care, mobile health components include monitoring, alerting, data collection, record maintenance, detection, and prevention systems.[6] Mobile health is defined as the application of mobile or wireless communication technologies to health and health care.[7] Mobile health services architecture include many settings, devices, and operational features—accessibility, timeliness, and integration (**Fig. 1**). Technology is a "practice extender" by performing some of the tasks others did to integrate

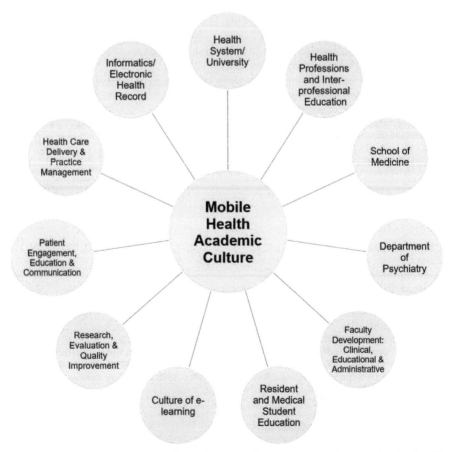

Fig. 1. How mobile health, smartphone/device, and apps integrate information in the digital age.

care[8]—indeed, it is considered a veritable team member.[9] Mobile health is used clinician to clinician, clinician to patient, and people to any others; the people and/or patient may be mobile or stationery.

Similar to telepsychiatry,[10] clinicians need a mobile health framework and skills and competencies and to meet needs of consumers, patients, caregivers, and other providers related to technology.[11–13] Mobile health may alter communication, boundaries, and privacy and confidentiality,[14] so clinicians are encouraged to screen what patients are using and help them use the "right" technology at the "right" time (eg, not using an app or text to express suicidal ideation). Similarly, it is important to evaluate apps to see if they are evidence-based and to use them in an evidence-based fashion.

There are a number of faculty development issues with mobile health, SP/D and apps—much like the case for social media competencies. The current generation of medical educators may not be as familiar with technology as much as the trainees, so bridging that gap must be done purposefully. This articles helps with reference to mobile health, SP/D, and app competencies so the reader can:

1. Have an outline of the competency-based medical education movement for competencies from telepsychiatry to social media to mobile health,
2. Grasp mobile health's components, concepts, operations, and processes, in comparison with in-person care, telepsychiatry and other technologies like social media,
3. Organize competencies for mobile health, SP/D, and apps using the Accreditation Council of Graduate Medical Education (ACGME) framework, and
4. Learn a basic approach to align teaching and evaluation with skill and patient outcomes for clinicians, departments and health care systems.

OVERVIEW OF COMPETENCIES IN MEDICINE, TELEPSYCHIATRY, AND OTHER TECHNOLOGIES

The Institute of Medicine's core competencies for the health professions include the ability to provide patient-centered care, work in interdisciplinary teams, use evidence-based practice, engage in quality improvement practices, *and* use information technology.[5] Competency-based medical education focuses on clinical skill development and curricula produce desired outcomes for learners rather than knowledge acquisition.[15] Learner-centered educational outcomes are set and teaching and assessment methods require alignment.[16,17] Faculty assessment of learners during patient care in addition to seminars ensures skill development.[17,18]

A straightforward competency framework is needed for technologies for faculty, program directors and administrators. The most common US framework is by the ACGME, which uses 6 domains: patient care, medical knowledge, practice-based learning and improvement, systems-based practice, professionalism, and interpersonal skills and communication.[18] Another useful framework is the Royal College Canadian Medical Education Directives for Specialists, which uses 7 roles that all physicians play: medical expert, communicator, collaborator, manager, health advocate, scholar, and professional.[19]

Other Technology Competencies

The telepsychiatry framework provided competencies, aligned standard andragogy/pedagogy methods for teaching and assessment, and highlighted faculty development issues.[10] It used a 3-level skill gradation rather than the Dreyfus model of learners with 5 levels[20]:

- Novice/advanced beginner (eg, early clinicians and/or those unfamiliar with technology);
- Competent/proficient (eg, able to translate in-person to technology-based care well); and
- Expert (eg, advanced in clinical care and via technology).

Telepsychiatry is similar to in-person care with patients and clinicians connecting synchronously (ie, in time), but a few significant and many minor adjustments in the clinical history (ie, interviewing, assessment, and treatment) and administration (eg, documentation, electronic health record [EHR], medicolegal issue, billing, and privacy/confidentiality).

The social media and networking competencies[21,22] provide a preview of how mobile health's asynchronous components may be approached. Social media may be defined as web-based and mobile services that allow people to share a connection, monitor progress, and create and manipulate text, audio, photos, and videos.[23] It poses substantial challenges compared with in-person and telepsychiatric care, such as:

1. It is asynchronous not synchronous, so it cannot be "organized" or structured like traditional care;
2. It may affect the therapeutic frame and create additional boundary issues;
3. It is conducted over public, private, and health system sites, making the data integration and security difficult, if not impossible;
4. Users overlap personal and professional life experiences, which causes complications similar to e-mail and texting; and
5. Clinicians cannot assume folks are who they state they are...there is a need to verify the identity of the patient for a social media account.[11]

A COMPETENCY-BASED FRAMEWORK FOR MOBILE HEALTH, SMARTPHONE/ DEVICE, AND APPS

Mobile health recontextualizes health care using mobile communication devices with mobile phones, tablet computers, wearable devices such as smart watches, and sensors.[24] As such, mobile health intersects with the field of remote patient monitoring of patients outside of conventional clinical settings (eg, at home for chronic disease management). Therefore, persons, patients, caregivers, and family members have more support if a problem arises and fewer emergency department visits and hospitalizations.

In era of health care, a physician or a patient can easily enter information (eg, appointment schedule), access it (eg, EHR) and make decisions anytime via a traditional desktop or his/her mobile personal computer, tablet, or SP/D. Mobile apps offer (1) portability for access anytime/anywhere, regardless of patient geography and transportation barriers; (2) an inexpensive option vs traditional desktop computers; and (3) additional features like context-aware interventions and sensors[25] with real-time feedback.

Similarities and Differences Between Mobile Health, Telepsychiatry, and Social Media

Mobile health is similar to in-person and telepsychiatric care, mainly because it is synchronous *and* anytime/anywhere—conceivably organized in a 24-hour, 7 days a week framework. This is similar to the Holter monitor in cardiology, which collects and transfers data, although those data are read intermittently and/or at the end of the data collection; therefore, it may be seen as asynchronous. Mobile health is different than in-person and telepsychiatric care in a few ways. First, because many professionals often use the same SP/D for professional and personal life, mobile health is "live" around the clock. In addition, patients increasingly have clinicians' telephone numbers. Finally, people are cued to respond to alerts on SP/Ds such that intervisit contacts may reset expectations if clinicians may receive and respond to messages.

Mobile health and social media and networking have common elements. Not all patients may be suitable for mobile health and social media (eg, impulsivity, disclosing too much per poor boundaries, failing to understand the medium). In contrast, they may provide a wraparound approach to life, similar to case managers for community schizophrenics.[11] They are outside the clinical visit, but may affect the therapeutic frame and create additional boundary issues—like the spontaneous, disruptive use of texts. But if the clinician helps the patient to use 1 app in a (structured) way that feeds into the EHR—instead of a half dozen apps that do not—the process is simplified, privacy is protected, and clinical decision making is improved (eg, using an app weekly for monitoring of depression).

Unique Features of Mobile Health

The mobile health devices (see **Fig. 1**) have the following features[26]:

- Voice/video calling: a convenient way for clinicians and patients to remotely communicate;
- Short message services and multimedia message services: transmit text messages and video clips/sound files as a cost-effective way to deliver education;
- Multimedia functions: provide a range of learning opportunities;
- Inbuilt sensors: touch, motion, and GPS sensors that simplify clinical assessment and lifestyle and social activities; and
- Device connectivity: practical and less error-prone data entry than manual processes.

Mobile health also has clinical decision support (CDS) and information flow management features. CDS provides clinicians, patients, and others with knowledge and person-specific information, intelligently filtered or presented at appropriate times, to enhance health and health care.[27] This technology improves patient outcomes, reduces unnecessary mistakes and expenses, and increases efficiency.[28] CDS is often seen as part of clinical informatics, but it is a key part of graduate medical education and lifelong learning.[29]

The Conceptual and Consensus Approach to the Mobile Health Competencies

This framework was built on an extensive review of the literature on teaching and learning, as well as on expert opinion, and uses the ACGME framework. We reviewed publications in Pubmed/Medline, using the key terms mobile health, apps, mental health, smartphones, competency, teaching, faculty development, medical education, and other terms mentioned in the article. We also hand searched the abstracts and indices of the articles we culled.

Expert option was solicited in 4 ways:

1. A series of medical educator conference calls focused on teaching competencies—for example, the conference calls series were composed of 2 groups of 8 medical educators from the United States and Canada to discuss educational competency development;

2. Discussion during several regional and national presentations (eg, American Association for Directors of Psychiatry Residency Training); for example, the participants included educational leaders (eg, course/program directors, chairs, deans, a national society executive director), educational researchers;
3. Individual discussions with educational and technological experts[13,14]—for example, those experienced in health services, mobile health, technology (eg, mobile health, SP/D. and apps), medicine, and informatics;
4. Input from national behavioral health organizations—for example, psychiatry/medicine, psychology, social work, counseling, marriage/family, psychiatric nursing, behavioral analysis)—via 2 rounds of input for the consensus process.[10,21]

Overall, a modified Delphi process[30] was used to develop an initial framework of areas (**Fig. 2**) based on qualitative analysis of identified themes. Then the themes were organized into competencies using the ACGME Milestones and the Royal College Canadian Medical Education Directives for Specialists roles.[18,19]

Mobile Health, Smartphones and Other Devices, and Apps Competencies

The patient care competency mainly includes history taking, engagement, interpersonal skills, assessment, education, management, and treatment planning

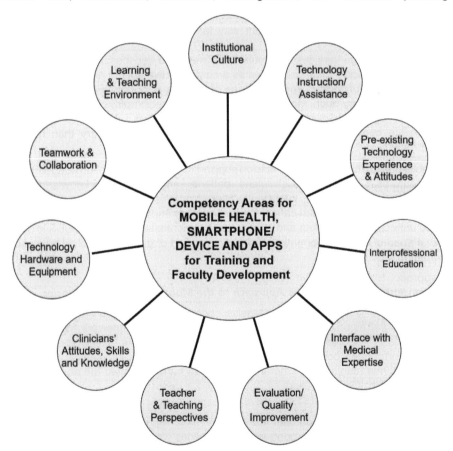

Fig. 2. Competency areas in mobile health, smartphone/device, and apps for training and faculty development.

(**Table 1**). It also includes administration, documentation, and medicolegal issues such as privacy, confidentiality, safety, data protection and integrity, and security. Clinicians should help patients to reflect on the pros and cons of mobile health, SP/D, and apps use as part of ongoing treatment and document these encounters (eg, as part of the consent form or in a progress note). This process may include, but is not be limited to, the competent or proficient clinician selecting the SP/D option based on patient preference, skill, and need (ie, purpose), as well as selecting the CDS tool option based on patient need, clinical purpose, and weighing the pros and cons of comparison apps. She or he may also find it helpful to know if the patient uses SP/D and apps for personal life, health care, and/or mental/behavioral health care, and seeing if the patient is aware of risks (eg, privacy, self-disclosure, potential for cyberbullying).

The patient care competency also included a subdomain for between visit data collection. Technology in the form of mobile health, SP/D, and apps can be useful for overcoming many of the barriers to accurate assessment of day-to-day life, including habits (eg, smoking), mood changes (ie, depression), activity, and vital signs (eg, blood pressure). This work is called ecological momentary assessment, and it involves repeated sampling of naturalistic behaviors and experiences.[31,32] A review of the topic discussed how technology methods have evolved from paper-and-pencil diary methods (eg, medication calendars) so that SP/Ds capture immediate self-reports by alarms (ie, signal dependent), within-person trajectories, and temporal sequences of behavior.[11] Changes in mood or affect therefore correlate better with clinician-rated affective symptoms and the subsequent risk of suicidal ideation in bipolar patients.

TEACHING, ASSESSMENT, AND EVALUATION OF MOBILE HEALTH, SMARTPHONES AND OTHER DEVICES, AND APPS

The outcome (ie, competency skill or behavior) should predetermine its measurement as well as teaching, supervision, and organization of clinical services. The supervisor's approach requires many things, including a plan for information flow and decisions and, if applicable, procedures for contact after hours. Initial, ongoing (ie, monitoring), and longitudinal documentation is needed (eg, consent form; progress notes). Patient requests for nonphone contact between visits (eg, apps, texts, e-mails) are increasing and this may not be a good regular practices and expectations for many patients.

Clinical Supervision of Mobile Health, Smartphones and Other Devices, and Apps Competencies

An approach to teaching these competencies involves a wide range of methodologies, settings, and participants (**Table 2**). Contacts with the patient throughout the week are best funneled into scheduled supervision as part of a caseload or quickly dealt with by a curbside consultation in real time. Time to reflect, consider options, and get advice before responding is suggested owing to clinical, administrative (ie, policies) and other ramifications. Trainees' work related to the patient care (eg, high-risk behaviors) and communication competencies can be aligned with teaching methods for clinical care with p and professional reflection, monitoring, and hygiene related to patient care and supervision (see **Table 2**). For example, a resident decided to add an app to track a veteran's mood because soldiers prefer to complete psychometric measures (eg, depression screening questionnaire) by iPhone rather than paper or computer owing to its interface, portability, and convenience.[11] However. an urgent issue arose, when an app transfer indicated new suicidal ideation. The trainee had to decide what to do: nothing (if it is a chronic behavior), e-mail, text, telephone call,

Table 1
A framework for faculty and trainee competencies for mobile health, smartphone/device and apps

Area/Topic	Novice/Advanced Beginner (ACGME Milestone Level 1–2)	Competent/Proficient (ACGME Milestone Level 3–4)	Advanced/Expert (ACGME Milestone Level 5)
Patient care			
History taking	Standard history and basic screen Are you using an SP/device and/or apps and for what? What for? Exercise? Entertainment? Social reasons? Health care?	Reflect on pros/cons of use and better screen Which SP/device and/or apps do you use? Use more/less than other technologies (e-mail, Internet, social media? Use SP/device and/or apps for health care: With your doctor, nurse or other staff? Share mental health (mental/behavioral health) issues? Aware of risks (eg, privacy, self-disclosure, time delays)?	Include SP/device and/or apps informed consent specifically Integrate details of personal and health care use into the history Discriminate types of personal use: significant other/spouse, friends, family; individual/group Screen for the patient use of privacy settings and provide advice
Engagement and interpersonal skills	Discuss impact of SP/device and/or apps use with others Incorporate SP/device and/or apps impact on professional life related to health care	Ask about preferences and how it/these influenced relationships with family, peers, and professional colleagues Consider how intimacy, emotion, and therapeutic relationship are affected Consider how it/these affect boundaries (see Professionalism)?	Provide guidance to patient and family on effective communication Instruct on impact of asynchronous vs synchronous communication methods Discuss expectations of parties

Assessment	Assess if use is important for personal life and/or health care Assess if SP/device and/or apps should not be used by a patient and document reason	Assess the healthy and unhealthy use in personal life and health care Consider the need for collateral info Integrate with overall in-person and longitudinal assessments Demonstrate flexibility and decide with the patient the role of SP/device and/or apps	Synthesize information from in-person TP, SP/device, and/or apps and other methods (including discordant data) Train, supervise, and consult to optimize assessment Identify pros/cons of using SP/device and/or apps and for what purpose(s)
Management and treatment planning	Integrate SP/D and/or apps into biopsychosocial approach Weigh pros/cons of decision support tool or app (see CDS in Knowledge) Monitor ongoing use and document memorable and problematic events If reasonable, focus part of a visit on the use of SP/device and/or apps and other technologies to talk in depth	Select option based on patient preference, skill (ie, purpose) (see Knowledge CDS) App to monitor mood Capture day-to-day accurate accounts of emotions, functioning, and activity Integrate the use of SP/device and/or apps on one treatment goal to monitor and engage Identify safety and other risk factors of use Triage complex, urgent/emergent issues to in-person care Research and apply tools (CDS Knowledge)	Select best mode for a given task: SP/device and/or apps, e-mail/text, telephone, and/or in person For medication issues: be aware of legal, billing and jurisdictional issues Research and disseminate procedures to prevent problems and manage clinical and administrative issues Advise on specific mental/behavioral health problems and specific patient populations with relative/absolute contraindications
Administration and documentation	Adhere to clinic, health system and professional requirements for in-person care Seek supervision and advice if needed	Develop standard language for these technologies for consent form, treatment plan and progress notes, particularly for nonroutine telepractice; seek consultation	Instruct on in-person, TP and SP/device, and/or apps applications related to documentation, privacy, and billing

(continued on next page)

Table 1
(continued)

Area/Topic	Novice/Advanced Beginner (ACGME Milestone Level 1–2)	Competent/Proficient (ACGME Milestone Level 3–4)	Advanced/Expert (ACGME Milestone Level 5)
Medicolegal issues: privacy, confidentiality, safety, data protection/integrity and security	Identify and adhere to relevant laws and regulations in the practice jurisdiction(s) of patient Clarify public or private access (ie, in EHR Communicate and data privacy (eg, email within EHR not Gmail)	Apply in-person relevant laws and regulations in any/all jurisdiction(s) to these technologies and adjust clinical care Educate patient about existing laws and adapt if none exist Obtain clinical and/or legal advice, as applicable	Teach/consult on in-person laws and regulations applied to technologies Develop legal and regulatory strategies (eg, emergencies) Update and consult with regulatory boards and health authorities
Interpersonal and communication skills			
Communication	Be flexible in discussing use Discuss problems if they arise with asynchronous options and arrange alternative options Seek advice on merit and method of responses, to patients	Discuss scope of communication, clarify expectations and anticipate problems (eg, feasibility of checking mobile health device off-site) Educate patient about pros/cons of asynchronous options Make brief, clear communications	Identify and trouble-shoot communication issues (eg, multiple meanings of acronyms, abbreviations and such communication) Educate/consult to colleagues about asynchronous technology use
Evaluation and feedback	Use evaluation parameter(s) for decision making and care Review examples with learner/supervisor	Adjust regular evaluation parameter(s) to incorporate real-time examples Coreview of others' examples of communication with learner/supervisor	Role model application of in-person skill to synchronous and asynchronous (ie, mobile health) technologies Develop and oversees in situ examples
Culture, diversity and special populations	Recognize culture impacts use and other trends in populations (eg, generation Y, autism spectrum)	Consider preferences and other implications of use and preference (eg, adolescent, veteran with posttraumatic stress disorder)	Instruct on cultural variations and how to adapt assessment and management approaches according to differences

Professionalism

Attitude	Be flexible and open to learning / Role model reflection / Consider all sources of information on decisions	Understand, educate and evaluate how use affects communication, relationship building, spontaneity, and quality / Role model willingness to engage improve	Provide leadership to colleagues on organizational policy or curricula for SP/device and/or apps and professionalism
Integrity and ethical behavior	Adhere to professional and governmental guidelines / Recognize boundary issues / Attend to privacy, confidentiality and professional boundaries	Weigh the pros and cons of use and data transfer with clinical and ethical principles / Reflect on personal vs professional contexts and microboundary and macroboundary violations (eg, texting patient after hours)	Role model, teach/consult others to manage complicated ethical issues for practice and professional identity / Research and develop approaches maintain therapeutic relationship
Scope and therapeutic objective(s)	Attend to in-person scope issues and observe for changes / Keep shared primary objective	Practice within scope and educate patient within license and standards (eg, Federal Trade Commission substantiation rule)	Teach/consult on in-person and technology adaptations and follow legal regulatory and fiscal issues

Systems-based practice

Interprofessional education	Learn/teach about technologies, and share information with others	Discuss specific issues for patients with team members for care and communication	Teach/consult to interprofessional education teams on/roles and practices; give feedback
Safety (see Patient care and professionalism)	Educate patient to call and/or set up additional appointment for emergencies / Seek consultation, when needed	Prevent, identify and stratify risk based on history (eg, not good for treatment plan) / Use in-person/synchronous (eg, video, telephone) methods for urgent issues	Adjust risk and its management to specific technology and instruct others in pitfalls in health care
Mobile health system practice	Incorporate and integrate data into workflow with technology (eg, EHR, desktop, portable)	Advise administration on (in) efficiencies, / Use sensors, remote monitors and other devices across sites (eg, home)	Use individual consult as an opportunity for building ongoing relationship / Integrate data into care

(continued on next page)

Table 1
(continued)

Area/Topic	Novice/Advanced Beginner (ACGME Milestone Level 1–2)	Competent/Proficient (ACGME Milestone Level 3–4)	Advanced/Expert (ACGME Milestone Level 5)
	Communicate and send data privately (eg, not Gmail)	Use EHR to collect and organize data and implement evidence-based decisions	Instruct on home health options to enhance evaluation and treatment
Practice-based learning			
Evaluation approach	Use global evaluations from patients, team and clinic about in-person and technology-based care	Be aware that in-person and other technologies have similarities/ differences Develop/promote attitudes and skills for consistency and quality of evaluation	Teach/consult on practice standards Compare/contrast information across professions and states/governments Shift policies and procedures
Quality improvement	Participate in chart review, case/ morbidity and mortality conference and other activities related to in-person and technology-based care	Apply/adapt in-person quality improvement principles to adjust assessment and/or care Educate participants on technology-specific principles and measures	Develop strategies to adhere and adapt in-person standards Teach/consult on how to analyze, select and evaluate quality improvement options
Learning, and teaching practices	Add technology-based learning opportunities to regular activities Consider role of technology in care	Seek out technology-specific education Develop additional technology-specific education in the short and/ or long term	Determine best context(s) for teaching and learning (eg, supervision, seminar/case conference)
Technology			
Adapt to technology	Use basic etiquette Identify differences between care in-person, TP, SP/device, and/or apps Clarify/spell out communications	Acknowledge issues and engage the patient (eg, can depressed patient use an app?) Prevent, identify and manage barriers, obstacles and miscommunications Learn to project self and express empathy	Advise on communication: avoid humor, self-deprecatory remarks and jokes; ways to express empathy Analyze what happens and make adjustments for next time

Technology operation	Pilot 1 or 2 SP/device and/or apps with peers to learn communication options	Gain experience with SP/device and/or apps Navigate options, if needed, and advise patients relative to goal and purpose	Research/teach/consult on approaches for clinical quality (eg, hard/software; accessories; trouble shooting)
Knowledge			
Definition of SP/device and/or apps	Recall definition of mobile health, SP/device and/or apps Name 2 or 3 mobile health, SP/device and/or apps with pros and cons	Define mobile health, SP/device and/or apps and various uses and risks/benefits to patients Professional skill with 2–3 SP/device and/or apps and a mobile health platform	Teach multiple SP/device and/or apps varieties; consults with colleagues Instruct on the approach to mobile health, selections of apps and pros and cons
Evidence base	Know basic dos and don'ts	Know if an app is evidence-based and used in an evidence-based clinical approach	Teach/consult to colleagues on best practice guidelines
Problem solving and prevention	Recognize and report problems Explain ways to better learn how to use an SP/device and/or apps product	Evaluate new products' and options' pros and cons Diagnose complex problems and/or resolve nonroutine problems that affect team Request/provide technical assistance	Research and disseminate information on platforms and latest developments (eg, privacy)
Decision support	Understand the ability of technology to help decision making Use for decision making and care Review examples with learner/supervisor	Find and evaluate ability of mobile health, SP/device and/or apps to help in decision making Compare the pros/cons for manual operations (eg, errors, duplications) Use for and adjust decision support	Advise/teach colleagues on how to evaluate decision support tools Instruct on fundamentals of adjusting to SP/device and/or apps parameter(s) to aid in decision making
Risks of using SP/device and/or apps	Identify 1 potential patient and 1 provider risk of SP/device and/or apps use (ie, boundary or privacy violation)	Identify 2–3 patient and provider risks and prevent, mitigate or eliminate them (eg, use privacy settings; avoid self-disclosure; manage cyberbullying)	Demonstrate extensive knowledge of use and advise colleagues Anticipate common pitfalls and how to prevent/mitigate them

Technically, mobile health options may be synchronous although most are asynchronous, so that term is used.
Abbreviation: TP (video), telepsychiatry.

Table 2
Faculty development related to mobile health, smartphone/device, and apps clinical competencies: teaching, assessment, and evaluation methods

Teaching Method	Context(s)	Competency Domain(s) Addressed	Learner Assessment
Didactic teaching: Patient care and knowledge			
All methods	Dependent on venue/setting	Knowledge, patient care, systems-based practice, technology—primarily knowledge at the precompetency and competency levels	Tests: multiple choice and short answer questions Audience participation
Brief didactic	Clinical setting (eg, replace nonsecure with secure technology)	Focus: solve immediate question/dilemma (eg, privacy)	Application to context (eg, pretest and posttest) Written tests: multiple choice and short answer questions
Grand rounds or longer didactic	Classroom in person, by video, or webinar	Focus: engage/help learners contextualize day-to-day events and gain further education Focus: research, trends and relevance vs e-mail/and synchronous modes (eg, in-person, TP, or telephone) Focus: CDS	
Case-based learning for attitudes and skills			
Brief vignettes Complex, multistep cases	Individual, pair/share and problem- and/or team-based learning (eg, how to triage a patient who reports suicidal ideation on a questionnaire)	Patient care, system-based practice, technology—knowledge for all levels of competency Provide content knowledge and effective for developing attitudes and skills Focus: apply knowledge to real-life examples and complex clinical situations to develop steps of treatment/management plans (eg, emergency) Focus: effective for highlighting key asynchronous events that are between visits and/or after hours	Case-based written tests: multiple choice, pretests and posttests and/or short answer questions (eg, next best step is . . .) Oral presentation with preassigned case (like flipped classroom) or in session case

Clinical care with patients (see patient care in **Table 1**)

Observing faculty	Live patient interview in-person or TP (eg, initial evaluation) in which SP/device and/or apps issue arises, is screened for and/or the focus of the conversation	Patient Care, communication, systems-based practice, technology—primarily at the pre competency level Adjust attitudes and demonstrate complex skills by faculty role modeling Foci: develop skills to set realistic expectations and communicate unidirectionally vs bidirectionally Focus: inappropriate use (eg, emergency; after hours; suicidal ideation comments)	Evaluation supplemented by review of SP/device and/or apps and chart Research on trends with SP/device and/or apps Develop and disseminate policies for technologies to in-person care
Group observed or cointerviewing	Group interview in person or TP: take turns with assessment; group and supervisor feedback Can also use separate room or 1-way mirror	Patient care, communication, professionalism, technology and systems-based practice (eg, decision support)—precompetency and competency levels Focus: develop skills and apply knowledge to screen, evaluate and plan Focus: use group/discussion and reflection to explore scope of practice, professionalism and cultural factors	Mini clinical evaluation exercise completed by faculty on each learner and direct verbal feedback. Peer-recorded written evaluation; peer review

Professional reflection, monitoring, and hygiene related to patient care and supervision

Caseload-based self-reflection, presentation, discussion and decision making In time supervision in person or at a distance on a critical incident (eg, emergency)	Review of personal and professional use Compare/contrast How is professional image projected? Supervision about	Patient care, communication, systems-based practice, professionalism, technology—all levels of competency Effective for developing attitudes and skills	Oral presentation in supervision, group, or grand rounds Chart review of treatment plan for decision making Policy development, review, and adaptation

(continued on next page)

Table 2
(continued)

Teaching Method	Context(s)	Competency Domain(s) Addressed	Learner Assessment
	Purpose(s), outcomes and adjustments Patient errors for those ill-equipped to use Review unexpected events Suicidal ideation, HI, bullying and/ or aggressive or sexual overtone	Focus: synthesis in a complex case or pattern analysis across a population; adjust management plans Focus: evaluate reactions and meaning of events, including transference and countertransference Focus: assess systems- and population-level thinking, decision support, workflow and resource allocation Examples: prevent/manage boundary violations (eg, personal picture or video transferred; patient friends trainee on social media); help patient adherence Focus: engage emergency response systems including authorities for duty to warn	Peer and faculty feedback Follow-up report on interventions and impact Longitudinal, cumulative evolution of clinical skills and relationship Timeliness of supervision
Quality improvement, evaluation, and research			
Case write-ups Literature reviews Quality improvement presentation/ project with interprofessional team, informatics team and administration	Trainee and mentor submission for committee, conference presentation, and/or final report or publication Evidence-, measurement-, and population-based care; systems-	Systems-based practice, practice-based learning—all levels of competency Effective for developing attitudes and skills, but less so for gaining knowledge	Evaluation of literature search Evaluation of written synopsis Verbal presentation, discussion, and group feedback Peer, interprofessional, supervisor, and administrator feedback

Quality improvement-related (eg, length of stay, informatics) committee	level thinking and health planning/ resource allocation	Focus: synthesis of a case in the short and long term and application to other cases Focus: good introduction to administration, evaluation and policy-oriented factors (eg, advanced knowledge gaps) Focus: evaluate apps to see if they are outcome and evidence based; develop an approach to use them in an evidence-based fashion	
Role as educator			
Provide didactic sessions and participate in group and interprofessional learning sessions	Learner participates in or leads discussions on mobile health, SP/ device, and/or apps	Knowledge, technology, systems-based practice, practice-based learning—all competency levels Develop attitudes and skills more so than content knowledge Focus: learn to work with an interprofessional team and adapt communication to multiple people Focus: develop advanced skills, such as enhancing capacity in distance staff (eg, teaching to use technology, decision support tools) Focus: evaluate apps to see if they are evidence-based and develop and used in an evidence-based approach Focus: dissemination, establish community/culture of practice and outreach across institutions	Reflection journal for observation Questions by participants Evaluation forms completed by participants Feedback solicited from participants of interest (eg, content expert, training director, informatics director)

Abbreviation: TP (video), telepsychiatry.

and/or trigger an emergency response. A text may be considered surprising in this context, but with personalization, caring sentiments, and a polite message, it may be therapeutic and successfully prevent worsening. Reflection, peer advice, and/or faculty supervision may be required quickly, which may necessitate on-site on-call or faculty of the day supervision, but they may triage this very differently than the trainee's ongoing supervisor. Regardless of the outcome, follow-up teaching methods of case presentation and/or a quality improvement project may help others to learn and investigate how a clinic can move forward.

A patient care and knowledge competency (eg, CDS) can be aligned with teaching methods for same, as seen in patient care and knowledge (see **Table 2**). For example, a resident decided to use attendance notifications to communicate with a depressed outpatient, caregivers, and other social supports. Over 3 months, it did not work, even though the depression had apparently started to lift with medication initiation and supportive therapy. The faculty supervisor reviewed the treatment plan, which was in order, but suggested to combine it with a tool for remote psychoeducation with motivational suggestions and personalized supportive messages.[33] This suggestion led to an occasional homework assignment[34] and, although the mood had not improved, the augmented treatment plan was helping.

Case-based learning (see **Table 2**) is a good teaching and learning method which uses real life examples or vignettes in seminar, site-based case conference and/or quality improvement/grand round presentations. It is important to draw from trainees' own experience with patients about mobile health, SP/D, and apps. Interactive methods like role plays can be used for flushing out the issues, to practice communication skills, identify options for decisions, and propose solutions for patients. The context for other settings and in-depth learning occurs through group input and feedback from peers and faculty. Furthermore, this provides an opportunity to build and/or solidify the resident role as an educator in teaching others (see **Table 2**).

MOBILE HEALTH IMPLICATIONS FOR ACADEMIC HEALTH CENTERS
Challenges for Clinicians and Systems

Traditionally, clinicians depend on research and clinical measures for care, so better customized measures for technologies are needed. Evidence-based guidelines for apps stratify purposeful use, content/process, measurement/assessment, and quality,[35,36] although app quality varies.[37] The Healthcare Information and Management Systems Society has created assessment guidelines for mobile technologies.[38] Current guidelines on e-mail, social media, and other technologies, however, are essentially just suggestions for clinicians integrating technology into practice.[10,14,21,22]

Faculty Development

Faculty and trainees are instruments of organizational change. Trainees teach faculty about the latest mobile health, SP/D, app, social media, Internet education websites, and other technologies. They inspire faculty—particularly through quality improvement and scholarship and research projects (eg, writing project, copresentations). Program evaluation uses quality improvement to meet patient (ie, Joint Commission, reimbursement), training, and other standards. It requires a philosophical approach, from seeing what happens with planned services to planning the outcomes and then designing the services—in advance. A grant may also facilitate system changes related to technology use (eg, an Institute of Medicine as a Profession and the Josiah Macy Jr. Foundation 2-year grant on social media).

Clinicians and faculty are at the crux of these paradigm shifts because they lead teams, provide care, and supervise trainees. One disturbing study revealed that students' digital professionalism deteriorated during core clinical clerkships, as measured by behavior, privacy, and attitudes.[39] Although today's clinicians and health care leaders and decision makers espouse, support, and drive innovation, they may also inadvertently stifle progress with inaction, conservative approaches (not to be confused with true incremental change), and resistance to change.

A Change in Culture Related to Technology, Training, and Patient Care

Many believe the academic psychiatry and medicine facilitate much of the change to technological innovation in the digital age, but many things like this get left behind to competing demands, inadequate resources, and/or higher priorities like patient care, training, and research.[40,41] Indeed, clinicians, leaders, and other stakeholders may not see mobile health, SP/D, and apps as central to the clinical care mission. Technology is significantly shaping people's lives and they have expectations in health care. Undergraduate universities, business,[42] banking, and even dating firms learned that, to survive, they had to adjust to people's preferences for electronic and online modalities. Businesses readily address change to remain viable and find new markets.[42,43] Medicine and business have one thing in common: the need to understand the person who is the patient or customer, their needs, and their behavior.[2,44]

New paradigms that integrate information technology, business, and medicine,[10,45] and are guided by institutional competencies and change management,[10] are needed. This process ensures that the technological infrastructure is in place, evidence based, supported by policy environment, and overall provides value-added clinical, education, and research interactions. For mobile health, SP/D and apps, there are at least 6 paradigm shifts at hand:

1. Patients and trainees of the X, Millennial/Y, and Z generations want and expect a digital health care experience[21,22];
2. Technology-based health care is different in some ways, but is at least as efficacious (eg, telepsychiatry) as in-person care and it leverages resources much more efficiently[46];
3. Health care systems must shift from a focus on knowledge to skills/competencies and then measure, evaluate and certify attainment to ensure the quality, safety, and efficiency of care[10,15,16];
4. Health care systems need an e-platform with information systems and technologies (eg, EHR, multiple entry portals via mobile health) as a foundation for "good" clinical care[10];
5. The mobile health paradigm is—and this may be the hardest part to see—a completely different, new and strategic way to frame health care—it may be staggeringly better and develop health care in completely new ways[11,45]; and
6. Financing and reimbursement streams (eg, the Center for Medicare and Medicaid Services) are beginning to reasonably let go of constraints and facilitate this change.[47]

Limitations to this set of mobile health and app competencies include that a broader consensus, with experts across organizations and fields of medicine (eg, American Medical Association, American Psychiatric Association, American Telemedicine Association). Second, the metrics of a more detailed approach to evaluation need to be spelled out; all competencies need to be measurable. Third, for both cross-sectional and longitudinal trajectories, with qualitative and quantitative evaluation of participants is suggested to iteratively improve the process. Finally, research is needed on organization change with technology and how a paradigm shift like mobile health recontextualizes digital health care.

ACKNOWLEDGMENTS

The authors would like to acknowledge the following organizations: the American Association of Medical Colleges, Accreditation Council of Graduate Medical Education, American Psychiatric Association Committee on Telepsychiatry, American Telemedicine Association and the Telemental Health Interest Group, Department of Psychiatry and Behavioral Sciences, University of California, Davis School of Medicine, Northern California Veterans Health Care System and Mental Health Service.

REFERENCES

1. Tachakra S, Wang X, Istepanian RS, et al. Mobile e-health: the unwired evolution of telemedicine. Telemed J E Health 2003;9(3):247–57.
2. Frydman GJ. Patient-driven research: rich opportunities and real risks. J Particip Med 2009. Available at: http://ojs.jopm.org/index.php/jpm/article/view/28/18. Accessed December 15, 2018.
3. World Health Organization. Telemedicine opportunities and developments in member states. Results of the second global survey on eHealth. Geneva (Switzerland): WHO Press; 2011.
4. Institute of Medicine. The core competencies needed for health care professionals. In: Health professions education: a bridge to quality. Washington, DC: The National Academies Press; 2003. https://doi.org/10.17226/10681. Accessed May 30, 2019.
5. Institute of Medicine. Health professions education summit. Available at: https://www.ncbi.nlm.nih.gov/books/NBK221516/. Accessed May 30, 2019.
6. Silva BMC, Rodrigues JPC, de la Torre I, et al. Mobile-health: a review of current state in 2015. J Biomed Inform 2015;56:265–72.
7. Steinhubl SR, Muse ED, Topol EJ. Can mobile health technologies transform health care? JAMA 2013;310:2395–6.
8. Raney L, Bergman D, Torous J, et al. Digitally driven integrated primary care and behavioral health: how technology can expand access to effective treatment. Curr Psychiatry Rep 2017;19(11):86.
9. Hilty DM, Sunderji N, Suo S, et al. Telepsychiatry/telebehavioral health and integrated care: evidence-base, best practice models and competencies. Int Rev Psychiatry 2019;1:1–18.
10. Hilty DM, Crawford A, Teshima J, et al. A framework for telepsychiatric training and e-health: competency-based education, evaluation and implications. Int Rev Psychiatry 2015;27:569–92.
11. Hilty DM, Chan S, Torous J, et al. New frontiers in healthcare and technology: Internet- and web-based mental options emerge to complement in-person and telepsychiatric care options. J Health Med Inform 2015;6:1–14.
12. Chan S, Torous J, Hinton L, et al. Towards a framework for evaluating mobile mental health apps. Telemed J E Health 2015;21:1038–41.
13. Hilty DM, Maheu M, Drude K, et al. Telebehavioral health, telemental health, e-therapy and e-health competencies: the need for an interdisciplinary framework. J Technol Behav Sci 2017. https://doi.org/10.1007/s41347-017-0036-0.
14. Maheu M, Drude K, Hertlein K, et al. An interdisciplinary framework for telebehavioral health competencies. J Technol Behav Sci 2018. Available at: https://link.springer.com/content/pdf/10.1007%2Fs41347-018-0046-6.pdf.

15. Frank JR, Mungroo R, Ahmad Y, et al. Toward a definition of competency-based education in medicine: a systematic review of published definitions. Med Teach 2010;32(8):631–7.
16. Iobst WF, Sherbino J, Ten Cate O, et al. Competency-based medical education in postgraduate medical education. Med Teach 2010;32(8):651–6.
17. Snell LS, Frank JR. Competencies, the tea bag model, and the end of time. Med Teach 2010;32(8):629–30.
18. Accreditation Council on Graduate Medical Education, 2013. Common Program Requirements. Available at: https://www.acgme.org/acgmeweb/Portals/0/PFAssets/ProgramRequirements/CPRs2013.pdf. Accessed May 30, 2019.
19. Royal College of Physicians and Surgeons, CanMEDS Framework, 2005. Available at: http://www.royalcollege.ca/portal/page/portal/rc/canmeds/framework. Accessed May 30, 2019.
20. Dreyfus SE, Dreyfus HL. A five-stage model of the mental activities involved in directed skill acquisition. Berkeley (CA): University of California, Operations Research Center; 1980. Available at: https://www.dtic.mil/cgi-bin/GetTRDoc?AD=ADA084551. Accessed May 30, 2019.
21. Hilty DM, Zalpuri I, Stubbe D, et al. Social media/networking as part of e-behavioral health and psychiatric education: competencies, teaching methods, and implications. J Tech Behav Sci 2018. https://doi.org/10.1007/s41347-018-0061-7.
22. Zalpuri I, Liu H, Stubbe D, et al. A competency-based framework for social media for trainees, faculty and others. Acad Psychiatry 2018;42(6):808–17.
23. Boyd DM, Ellison NB. Social network sites: definition, history, and scholarship. J Comput Mediat Commun 2008;13:210–30.
24. Torous J, Chan RS, Yee-Marie Tan S, et al. Patient smartphone ownership and interest in mobile apps to monitor symptoms of mental health conditions: a survey in four geographically distinct psychiatric clinics. JMIR Ment Health 2014;1:e5.
25. Kumari P, Mathew L, Syal P. Increasing trend of wearables and multimodal interface for human activity monitoring: a review. Biosens Bioelectron 2017;90:298–307.
26. Honeyman E, Ding H, Varnfield M, et al. Mobile health applications in cardiac care. Interv Cardiol 2014;6(2):227–40.
27. Osheroff JA, Teichc JM, Middletone B, et al. A roadmap for national action on clinical decision support. J Am Med Inform Assoc 2007;14:141–5.
28. Kawamoto K, Houlihan Ca, Balas EA, et al. Improving clinical practice using clinical decision support systems: a systematic review of trials to identify features critical to success. BMJ 2005;330:765.
29. Torous J, Chan S, Boland R, et al. Clinical informatics in psychiatric training. Acad Psychiatry 2017. https://doi.org/10.1007/s40596-017-0811-4.
30. Srinivasan M, Li ST, Meyers FJ, et al. Teaching as a competency for medical educators: competencies for medical educators. Acad Med 2011;86(10):1211–20.
31. Carlson EB, Field NP, Ruzek JI, et al. Advantages and psychometric validation of proximal intensive assessments of patient-reported outcomes collected in daily life. Qual Life Res 2016;25:507–16.
32. Van Os J, Delespaul P, Barge D, et al. Testing an mHealth momentary assessment Routine Outcome Monitoring application: a focus on restoration of daily life positive mood states. PLoS One 2014;9:e115254.
33. Gonzalez J, Williams JW, Noël PH, et al. Adherence to mental health treatment in a primary care clinic. J Am Board Fam Pract 2010;18:87–96.
34. Harrison V, Proudfoot J, Wee PP, et al. Mobile mental health: review of the emerging field and proof of concept study. J Ment Health 2011;20:509–24.

35. Gonnermann A, von Jan U, Albrecht UV. Draft guideline for the development of evidence based medicine-related apps. Stud Health Technol Inform 2015;210: 637–41.

36. Agarwal S, LeFevre AE, Lee J, et al. Guidelines for reporting of health interventions using mobile phones: mobile health (mHealth) evidence reporting and assessment (mERA) checklist. BMJ 2016;352:i1174.

37. Grundy QH, Wang Z, Bero LA. Challenges in assessing mobile health app quality: a systematic review of prevalent and innovative methods. Am J Prev Med 2016;51(6):1051–9.

38. Arellano P, Bochinski J, Elias B, et al. Selecting a mobile app: evaluating the usability of medical applications 2012. Available at: www.mhimss.org/sites/default/files/resourcemedia/pdf/HIMSSguidetoappusabilityv1mHIMSS.pdf. Accessed May 30, 2019.

39. Mostaghimi A, Olszewski AE, Bell SK, et al. Erosion of digital professionalism during medical students' core clinical clerkships. JMIR Med Educ 2017;3(1):e9.

40. Armstrong EG, Mackey M, Spear SJ. Medical education as a process management problem. Acad Med 2004;79:721–8.

41. Bowe CM, Lahey L, Armstrong E, et al. Questioning the "big assumptions." Part II: recognizing organizational contradictions that impede institutional change. Med Educ 2003;37(8):723–33.

42. Christensen CM. Disruptive innovation: can health care learn from other industries? A conversation with Clayton M. Christensen. Interview by Mark D. Smith. Health Aff (Millwood) 2007;26(3):w288–95.

43. Kotter J. Leading change. Boston: Harvard Business School Press; 1996.

44. Miles A, Mezzich J. The care of the patient and the soul of the clinic: person-centered medicine as an emergent model of modern clinical practice. Int J Pers Cent Med 2011;1:207–22.

45. Hilty DM, Uno J. Chan S, et al. Role of technology in professional development. Psychiatr Clin N Amer, in press.

46. Hilty DM, Ferrer D, Callahan EJ. The effectiveness of telemental health: a 2013 review. Telemed J E Health 2013;19:444–54.

47. Center for Medicare and Medicaid Services. Clinical decision support. Available at: https://www.cms.gov/Regulations-and-Guidance/Legislation/EHRIncentive Programs/Downloads/ClinicalDecisionSupport_Tipsheet-.pdf. Accessed December 15, 2018.

A Narrative on Career Transitions in Academic Psychiatry

Frederick G. Guggenheim, MD[a,b],*

KEYWORDS

- Transitions - Adult development - Academic career - Time management - Salaries
- Fitting in

KEY POINTS

- In addition to doing what one is hired for (research, teaching, patient care, administration), your career may well benefit from going the extra mile.
- Being familiar with departmental priorities will help you to suggest and carry out new initiatives consistent with those priorities.
- It is important to also know your own priorities.

STARTING AN ACADEMIC CAREER

Becoming an academic psychiatrist is surely a complex decision, based on the resident's or fellow's personal values. Other important components to the decision: interest in research or teaching; access to mentors and other valued role models; and absence of barriers, such as massive educational debt.[1] One key issue is that the academician will have her or his time commitments and financial reimbursement *somewhat* or *a lot* under her or his control, whereas the clinical practitioner will typically have time and money *mostly* under her or his control; both choices come with significant privilege in helping patients, the need to work well with others, and responsibility for individual lives and other social missions.

An academic career means being associated with a university, and as such, there is implied a willingness to support, and be supported by, a community of scholars. Some members of a department of psychiatry may be doing primarily research, some teaching, others primarily administration, still others patient care. Most will do a combination of these activities, with the goal of "keeping the (university) ship afloat" and aspiring to

Conflicts of Interest: The author has no commercial or financial conflicts of interest.
a University of Nebraska Medical Center College of Medicine, Omaha, NE, USA; b University of Arkansas for Medical Sciences, Little Rock, AR, USA
* 1500 Little Raven Street, #305, Denver, CO 80202.
E-mail address: guggenheimf@gmail.com

excellence. This differs considerably from a career in private practice, Veterans Health Administration (VHA), or a Community Mental Health Center (CMHC) practice, in which the goal is the provision of excellent service to patients. Some of these practitioners will do a small amount of teaching, or serve on committees of professional organizations, "keeping the (service community) ship afloat."

In commencing an academic career, the new faculty member must always ask fundamental questions such as: Am I in this new position merely as a job, or am I here as a career move? Is this job and this organization something that I crave to nourish, or is this just a vanity, a competition that I want to participate in? Do I need to make more money, and if so, according to whose needs? Do I like being in an organization, or do I really like more my own autonomy? How about the culture of the department? Is this a *publish or perish* organization, or a *publish and perish* culture? In the latter case, publishing and doing research was interpreted by a particular chair as implying that one was not paying enough attention to the department's priority of teaching.

Will I pinch myself in this new job: is this wonderful place for real? In the place where I will be working, will I really look forward to coming to work every day? Will I hurry to work, excited to be there? Am I going to make a significant contribution to the organization? Will I be adding to, or subtracting from, the organization? Will my new boss see me as an asset, or as a "pain in the butt"?

OBTAINING A FACULTY POSITION IN ACADEMIA

Will the new position fit with one's career goals? Will going to work each day be an answer to a dream? Will it fit in with family plans and needs? As Karen Leslie writes,[2] "academic and career development of faculty is paramount to the success of both individual faculty members and the institutions in which they work. This [support of] career development [should] begin during the transition from postgraduate or graduate training to faculty appointment, ... continues to retirement...[It] can support and promote the alignment of values and goals with the overall aim of facilitating career success and fulfillment."

Transition in academia means getting a job, or a better job, whether at the instructor's level, or at the chair's level. Some jobs are filled by openly soliciting specific candidates, others by ads. Rather than just saying breathlessly, "Yes!" to an offer, one needs to be well informed. Just as all coughs and all back pains are different, so all departments' funding and budget issues are different, too. These matters might impact one's decision to accept an offer, yet this information may be difficult to come by.

Salary ranges for instructor, assistant professor, associate professor, professor, and chair of psychiatry for various regions of the country are prepared by the American Association of Medical Schools with updates yearly, available to deans of all medical schools. Yet questioning about salaries of various faculty members during a recruitment visit is typically considered socially taboo. Starting salaries are almost always different from that of an established faculty member. Is the position permanent, or is it grant-dependent? Is it vacant due to the replacement of a faculty member? If so, does the reason given seem plausible or are there other issues? What discretionary perks are variable, what guaranteed? Is the medical school's annual budget dependent on the fiscal health of its state? Subspecialty certification will enhance salary in most academic positions.

State support of medical schools can vary widely from school to school, and sometimes from year to year. These fluctuations, though, rarely change salaries, but they may limit salary increases over time. State medical schools vary from 100% to partially state-supported to only minimally state-assisted. With state funding also may come the burdensome requirement to submit to state-required regulations for purchasing. Some private medical schools also receive a smaller amount of state funding without such requirements. Depending on the state's fiscal shape in a particular year, support from the state for the medical school and various medical school service programs can vary from year to year. These matters may, or may not, impact the dean's funding or the department's bottom line.

At Harvard, with its $37 billion endowment, there is an obscure but powerful mantra, "Each tub on its own bottom." This means that each school, and each department is essentially on its own. Of course, there is a specific allotment for the law school, the business school, and the medical school. But don't go looking for support just because of the massive endowment, for its distribution is highly formulaic and regulated by the president and the Board of Overseers. However, consider working with university philanthropy arms as a source of funding for special educational and research programs that tie to their mission and the community at large.

Initial recruiting packages vary widely concerning reimbursement to support the initial visit to the department, such as airfare, hotel, and meals. Some departments' initial visits are fully supported, some not at all. Some visits also depend on who is seeking who's help: if you apply for a regular position and there are few positions available, you have little leverage; on the other hand, if they need many people, you fill a much needed niche, and/or they recruit you, you have more leverage. Even early career psychiatrists may be able to receive help with loan reduction (eg, VHA Educational Debt Loan Repayment). Keep in mind, too, that packages include salary, benefits, and positions; some institutions' positions (eg, director of the clerkship) are more meaningful than the money.

When I was recruited to Massachusetts General Hospital (MGH), for my first postresidency job, it was before the department had established its organized private practice plan, its service contracts, pharmaceutical company money for drug research projects, and lucrative continuing medical education programs, although there were some National Institutes of Health grants. The department's financial support from the hospital and the medical school was mainly limited to full-time equivalents (FTEs) with little if any discretionary money. Hence, there was no help for my initial recruiting visit. However, I had a great decade there, learning the skills to be a teacher and discovering my interest in being an educator. Eventually the department branched out in areas that contributed to its bottom line, meaning backing for various recruiting and faculty development needs. Potential "dowries" for researchers for laboratory equipment and for ancillary personnel can vary from nothing to $50,000 to $50,000,000 depending on the dean's support and the department's research endowment.

Job Offers Can Vary Widely

It's not always about how attractive the candidate is. Departments may have constraints. Sometimes there is wiggle room, and sometimes not. During a recruitment visit, it's always wise to quietly figure out, if possible, what are the departmental financial issues. Candidates need to be informed and be selective. Always be gracious. There are sometimes more open slots than there are available candidates. But also bear in mind when negotiating, "You are unique, but are you unique enough?" This is a difficult decision for even the healthiest of egos.

The Faculty Package

Is it a good fit? More than just the job description, what about night call duties and the number of patients to be covered? Does the faculty practice plan aid or drive the department? Is there protected time for teaching or research? What about vacation time? Faculty morale? How about the initial salary and reimbursement for the moving van? Is there the availability of some administrative help for academic or service responsibilities? Critically important is the availability of senior faculty mentoring before and after attaining tenure. Finally, does there seem to be potential for advancement within the department?

Perks

Typically, the range for fringe benefits from one department to the next may vary between 10% and 22%. The business manager or administrator will know details. A recruitment candidate should try to see him or her on a second visit. Malpractice, disability, health, dental, and life insurance will be provided. About retirement plans: is there a departmental match for retirement contributions? Some schools require 5-year vesting before retirement plans can be moved to another job site. Is there support for a house down payment (California especially)? Is there money for membership in academic societies, travel to meetings and meeting registration fees? Is there financial assistance for college tuition for children?

The Area

Is there affordable real estate and a good fit for recreational activities? What about expected commuting time? Schools for children? Crucially important, what about employment opportunities for one's spouse, which may be limited in smaller cities?

CHOOSING THE DEPARTMENT AND DEVELOPING A PROSPEROUS CAREER

In the hiring process, the chair chooses the candidate, but the candidate is also choosing to work for him or her. It's always good to know essential information about one's new boss, who may have some control over one's working conditions and career advancement. My experience comes from being a departmental chair for 15 years, serving on the Executive Committee of the American Association of Chairs of Departments of Psychiatry for a dozen years, and serving as president as well.

When deciding on which department to choose during a journey of recruitment, it is useful to have had positive (and/or negative) role models of departments and chairs to compare and contrast. Chairs are responsible for beginning salary levels and then salary adjustments, based on clinical or scholarly productivity. Chairs also may have a hand in dispensing perks of all sorts and sometimes even appointments to desirable national committee assignments.

It is reasonable to ask about the chair's plans and the length of time past chairs have stayed, as well as where they went thereafter. Almost all chairs have at least 10-year plans of staying. Occasionally, some chairs move after just a few years because they have a chance to move their career forward and upward in the institution or at another institution. There seems to be a bell-shaped survival distribution, with a few chairs turning out to be not a good fit and leaving within 3 years, and another small group "covered with Teflon," lasting decades.

Prospering and Advancing One's Career

In addition to doing what one is hired for (research, teaching, patient care, administration), your career may well benefit from some or all of the following:

- Going the extra mile
- Suggesting and carrying out new initiatives consistent with departmental priorities

- Being successful at "managing up" and "managing down" within the department
- Knowing promotion criteria, which may differ from department to department
- Acting as fits one's balanced life style (but there can be consequences if this impacts on what is expected from the projected job description)
- Having fun with other faculty members
- Being mentored within (and/or outside) the department
- Engaging in committee work within the department: it does help to keep the machine running
- Writing, writing, writing: by oneself or with others in the department or as a result of participating in working committees of national psychiatric organizations
- Giving talks (although they rarely count for promotion and tenure)
- Becoming known outside the department, through serving on regional or national committees, even peer reviewing journals, because promotion to associate or full professor in many departments requires that you be known regionally or nationally.

Finally, time management is an essential skill. One esteemed faculty member, rising to full professor at Harvard, returned a paper I had given him to critique with the annotation on the top of it, "Circling over Baltimore, 11:34 PM." Another aspiring faculty member told me that he could write his papers only when he was out of town: he did his best work in airplanes and hotels. Still another faculty member shared with me that his most productive times are in the mornings before the rest of the family has arisen. His colleague, also in the same consultation division, found that his best writing times were when everyone else in the house has gone to bed.

Another aspect of time management relates to having children. In higher education, for women this is sometimes referred to as the "Mommy Tenure Track."[3–5] (Although the term may seem initially pejorative, it is not intended that way.) Each institution has its own sets of rules, regulations, and "permissiveness," with time off for maternal leave, paternal leave, and time off the tenure clock for those so involved.

Helping the chair by being of service will be greatly appreciated and requires perspective and ability to put the department and institution missions first. Chairs need help, as much, if not more than, other departmental members. Being readily available to the chair for important assigned tasks is an important way to survive and flourish. Being able to focus on departmental needs: such as giving superb patient care, and respecting financial realities is also important. If requested, working well with the dean, the chancellor, and major department donors as appropriate, is certainly a plus.

Chairs do not need faculty to be a "pain in the butt," as occurs with some faculty members, perhaps due to their unresolved issues with past authority figures. It is important for the faculty member to know the difference between being a high maintenance and a low maintenance faculty member. It is key to be productive and helpful, because things may be difficult during any window of time due to loss of funding for a project or research or there is a downsizing, unexpectedly.

Being a Chair or Other Leader

Often the most helpful individuals for a new chair are the business manager/administrator and the chair's executive assistant, if both are long-standing members of the department, competent, and cheerful. Finances and personnel matters often consume much of the first years on the job. All division chiefs will be as helpful as possible, yet with their own agendas, of course.[6]

Another key aspect of being a chair is assessing strengths, weaknesses, and opportunities. The overall goal is to help the department, faculty, trainees, community, and the institution prosper. Strategic changes may well be needed. Examples: moving existing faculty around to positions that meet their real skill sets (research, teaching); regionally recruiting new faculty members to key medical student teaching positions to enhance residency recruitment; and building the private practice plan by setting realistic (and higher) goals.

Most chairs are good leaders, but some manage their responsibilities and interpersonal interactions much better than others. As psychotherapists, we are trained in issues of transference and countertransference with the individual patient. But transference toward the chair, both positive and negative, can be real, too. That is, the chair and his or her performance can be fairly rated, overrated (widely praised), or underrated (denigrated), based on any number of variables. The best chairs continue to be academically productive, move up in their organizations, and may have national positions. Many have added to their psychiatric career with business, leadership, and/or other training.

Developing relationships is key for a chair, and in my case, these were with institutional leaders at the state hospital and at the VA. They were interested in excellence, within the constraints of their budgets, but a dean can give funds for a number of vacant FTEs at the medical school to help develop these relationships. Alignment of missions with interests, in my case the Arkansas medical students' substantial interests in psycho-social aspects of life and psychiatry, facilitated recruitment into the residency program, but only after recruitment of excellent educators. Many parties, including senior faculty, valued the concept of a community of scholars, and this linked the department with philanthropists in the community, who could see both the need for, and value of, good psychiatry. This type of support of major initiatives makes building the department, a very demanding job, very rewarding!

But not all chair choices by the dean and his or her search committee work out well, for a variety of reasons. Although all chair-designates have both great CVs and good ability to "manage up" during their recruitment, not all chair-designates are good at "managing down," relating appropriately with their potential faculty, administrative staff, and major donors. Other new chairs, faced with burgeoning new responsibilities, are discovered to have poor time management skills, being constantly tardy in the submission of crucial financial reports, specific progress reports to the dean, promotion letters with deadlines, or signing off on grants and service agreements.

SUMMARY

In summary, being an academic psychiatrist means participating in a dynamic journey. But be aware, an academic career is usually associated with many transitions. Assuming this is a life-long sojourn, there will be numerous changes and unexpected challenges. Many organizations strive to give the *appearance of current stability*, with prospects for growth. But change within any organization is the rule, not the exception. There also will be *personal challenges* outside of academia, within the real world of money, moving, and medical maladies. Finally, there will also be *developmental changes within oneself*. George Engel's biopsychosocial model can well be applied here to the biological, psychological, and social changes and challenges that will occur over the career of an evolving psychiatrist.[7]

ODYSSEYS IN AN ACADEMIC LIFE

Many an academic career, with its odysseys and its developmental phases, often makes sense best in retrospect rather than in prospect. Although many academicians complete their careers within a single institution, still others do not. That is because some transitions in academia derive from chance and opportunity, favoring the prepared mind. Some academicians pursue their established goals relentlessly; others are startled to be able to follow unexpected opportunities. For example, some individuals "always" have wanted to be a chair; other chairs are surprised at entering that academic phase, whereas still other academics abhor administration.

How do these transitions happen? Unexpected openings occur. Unpredictably, an important mentor or collaborator leaves the institution. There are unplanned recruitment opportunities, impromptu meetings. A new chair devalues one's work. A mentor suggests a new career phase is appropriate.

Narrative of the Executive Director of the American Board of Psychiatry and Neurology

The life narrative of the Executive Director of the American Board of Psychiatry and Neurology is a good example of the unexpected twists and turns associated with a successful academic career, that only in retrospect seem most understandable.[8] Dr Faulkner underlines the fact that "others have had a major impact on all that I accomplished throughout my professional life." He graduated from the University of Washington School of Medicine, then a psychiatric residency in Arkansas. While there, he attended the Chief Residents Conference in Tarrytown where he met Jim Eaton, MD, Director of the Education Branch at the National Institute of Mental Health (NIMH). That led to Faulkner being selected to spend the last 4 months of his residency as an administrative fellow in the Psychiatric Education Branch at NIMH. There he met the incoming Commissioner of Mental Health for Arkansas, which facilitated his return to Arkansas as Deputy Commissioner for Community Mental Health Service. He stayed in Little Rock for another 2 years.

Then through established contacts while continuing to consult for the NIMH Branch, Falkner was recruited back to the northwest for a decade, where he was with the Oregon Health Sciences University as Residency Training Director, later Director of Education. From there, because of contacts, he was recruited to the University of South Carolina as Chair, later Interim Dean, then Dean of the School of Medicine for a total of 16 years. Thence, to the American Board of Psychiatry and Neurology as Executive Director, where he had previously been a director. At each twist of his early career, established mentors spotted his "going the extra mile" with excellence; later in more senior positions, his job performance illuminated his talents.

My Path and First Job

During my own postresidency, I had moves to Boston, then to Dallas, and on to Little Rock, thence to Providence in partial retirement, and finally to Denver. I was fortunate to have only superb academic chairs to work for. Uniformly they were friendly, accessible, and gave me good career advice at each phase of my development. But occasionally along the journeys of my career while I was still choosing a position, at some departments I heard disturbing tales about their chairs from disgruntled faculty.

With my first job at MGH, at an instructor level, then quickly rising to as assistant professor, I found that there was no wiggle room on salary or perks. But the department did need to build an office for me, in what had been an underutilized waiting room. I had a wonderful 10 years there as Director of the Private Psychiatric Consult

Service and Director of the Behavioral Science courses at MGH, neither position I held for my first 2 years.

Making a Change to a New Job

My next move was to Dallas as an associate professor and as the Director of the Psychiatric Consult Service. The reason that I initiated a search for this position after a decade was the realization that there would not be many opportunities for departmental growth at MGH due to my lower position in the very talented pecking order. After initiating a search that took me to many departments around the country, I found a best fit for me, due to the chair and an emerging department, good resources and a can-do department. At Southwestern Medical School, the University of Texas Health Science Center at Dallas, I was offered an acceptable salary and was able to establish the FTE parameters of the psychiatric consultation liaison faculty that I would join and supervise. Jokingly, I asked the chair for season tickets to the Cowboys' football games, only to learn, a bit later, that my chair was on close terms with the Cowboys' owner. Realizing this was an inappropriate request, I quickly, and embarrassingly, backed off. I had a great 6 years in Dallas.

How I Became a Chair

Even though I was comfortable and happy in my position, I was receiving several offers to go elsewhere. Even though being a chair was not part of my own long-term plan, I ended up being recruited to be a chair. The offer to look at this endowed chair was based on a friendship I made at an American Psychiatric Association Task Force that I set up to look at national funding issues for psychiatric consultation services. While negotiating with the University of Arkansas for Medical Sciences dean for my chair, I did not even mention my salary level, but asked for a number of potential FTEs that I could recruit for, and they were given. Later I realized that another candidate for the chair was turned away because all he negotiated for was for his laboratory and his collaborators, but nothing for the department. After a year, my salary was generously established at competitive levels for that region of the country. I had a great 15-year run as chair.

Ten years into the chair, at age 60, after a heart attack, I found I was not as interested or as interesting as chair, although I was still good at my job. After 5 more years post myocardial infarction, I stepped down as chair. Then a year later, I had a period of personal emotional turmoil due to the World Trade Center disaster of 9/11: "What is my life about? What is most important in this phase of my life? Where do I want to be when I die?" These questions arose even though we had no friends or associates who died at the World Trade Center.

Weighing Priorities of Life, Family, and Academia

But at age 70, my wife and I decided we still had another move left in us. We moved, this time for a place to live, because of family reasons. The job description was much less important this time. After 3 years in Providence, at an unaffiliated CMHC, with its dysfunctional management, I wanted to get back into academia. At the same time, fortunately, I was recruited to be a clinical professor at Brown Medical School and Associate Director of a Residents' Continuity Clinic. I served there for another decade. Then, at age 80, I retired and moved to Denver to be with other family. Now I continue to write, but at a very part-time level. Very recently, I've been appointed as an adjunct professor at the University of Nebraska Medical Center College of Medicine to consult with the chair.

LIFE CHANGES AND TRANSITIONS

During an academic career there will occur some or many of the following life changes or deflections: marriage or partnership, buying a house, childrearing, divorce, moving, leaving friends behind, remarriage, buying another house, moving, buying another house, children growing up, aging, one's own gradual physical disintegration, a malpractice suit, death of siblings, death of parents, death of friends, death of ambition, and last, dementia or chronic physical illness in oneself or one's spouse. Biology sometimes steps in. Any or all of these can have a profound impact for some individuals on what is important in one's life, one's career. Such transitions can collide with what is worth "going the extra mile" for. And to be successful in academia, "going the extra mile," proving that one is special for some aspect of "the organization," is important.

A key dimension of this are changes within oneself. During an evolving life, including an academic career, there are certain normative, developmental challenges that Erikson details.[9] I think these stages can be conceptually extended to encompass the career pathway of the academic psychiatrist. Erikson's[9] cyclical changes impact on one's intrapersonal life, and hence on career issues. He focused on these psychosocial transitions with age-defined tasks and crises. For the new, mid-career, and older faculty, their personal challenges can be centered in the realm of, respectively, *Loving, Caring, and Wisdom*:

- For the *younger faculty member*, tasks are *intimacy versus isolation.* Loving with dating, marriage or domestic partnership, family, and friendships are important. Those that have yet to, or fail to, form lasting relationships may feel isolated and alone.
- For the *mid-level faculty*, from age 40 on, tasks are *generativity versus stagnation.* There may be the move up the academic ladder, or the transition to private practice. By this age, faculty members are normally settled in their life and know what is important to them. They are engaged in caring. A person may enjoy raising children, participating in community/academic activities, and/or professional organizations that give a sense of purpose. If a person is not comfortable with the way life is progressing, he or she may feel useless.
- For the *older faculty member*, perhaps 65 on, often comes wisdom. This phase is the last chapter of an individual's academic life with retirement approaching. Tasks concern *ego integrity versus despair.* One deals with enduring comprehensiveness of one's values, including authenticity and integrating the past phases of one's life as one moves forward. Does the individual forge ahead or merely maintain, doing the same task (as she or he perceives it) day by day? It means acceptance of life in its fullness: what was accomplished, or not. Focusing on past failures leads to depression and hopelessness.

Actual retirement means many things to many people. The federal Age Discrimination Act was passed in 1986. For the next 8 years, until 1994, colleges and universities were granted an exemption that permitted them to continue mandatory retirement for the professoriate at age 70. Since then, age per se is not a disqualification for continuing on in academia. For one of my gurus, George Engel, MD, his mandatory retirement meant, for him, no longer serving on academic committees that weren't meaningful, but otherwise George continued on as before, as long as he was medically able. I am uncertain if his salary continued or not.

For some, being 65 or 70 now means continuing on as usual, but no more onerous night call. For others, voluntary academic retirement means *"rehirement,"* actively seeking out a new career or a new job, perhaps in a new place. Such individuals are taking advantage of good health and an adequate nest egg to be able to make another move, either major or minor. Others voluntarily choose to work part-time, at the same or a different place: with more time for hobbies and necessary medical visits. Still others who are working full-time, with flagging productivity, may be edged out, and for that reason, may not leave so willingly. Integrity versus despair can rear its head.

Many faculty members, accustomed to being active with leadership roles and writing, choose to replicate some of that pleasurable activity in full retirement. To be their good selves, they *feel* their authenticity by continuing to write academic papers; by taking classes in, for example, creative writing; by attending classes in art appreciation; and by serving on the executive director's advisory committee at an independent living facility. Finally, sometimes a retiree taking care of an ailing spouse would seem to take on the role of full-time or part-time work. In such instances, these retirees may feel fulfilled by their loving and caring; for others, without their own sense of loving to fall back on, despair can be nipping around the corner.

SUMMARY

The journey into academic psychiatry is a complex, meaningful, and exciting adventure. One should not see this as a solo trip: mentors can complement and augment the experience.

ACKNOWLEDGMENTS

The author thanks Art Paulson, PhD, Professor of Political Science Emeritus, Southern Connecticut State University; G. Richard Smith, MD, Marie Wilson Howells Professor and Chair, Department of Psychiatry, College of Medicine, University of Arkansas for Medical Sciences; Paul Lieberman, MD, Clinical Professor of Psychiatry at Alpert Medical School of Brown University; Richard Brandenburg, Dean and Professor Emeritus of Business Administration, University of Vermont; and Olivia Guggenheim, BA, for their valuable critiques of this article.

REFERENCES

1. Borges NJ, Navarro AM, Grover A, et al. How, when, and why do physicians choose careers in academic medicine? A literature review. Acad Med 2010;85: 680–6.
2. Leslie K. Faculty development for academic and career development. In: Steinert Y, editor. Faculty development in the health professions. New York: Springer; 2014. p. 97–118.
3. Draznin J. The "mommy tenure track." Acad Med 2004;79:289–90.
4. Kittelstrom A. The academic-motherhood handicap. Chron High Educ 2010.
5. Pololi LH, Jones SJ. Women faculty: an analysis of their experiences in academic medicine and their coping strategies. Gend Med 2010;7:438–50.
6. Kramer R, Mucha PJ. Five tips on surviving your first year as a department head. Chron High Educ 2018.
7. Engel GL. The clinical application of the biopsychosocial model. Am J Psychiatry 1980;137:535–44.
8. Faulkner LR. Personal reflections on a career of transitions. J Am Acad Psychiatry Law 2007;35:253–9.
9. Erikson EH. Childhood and society. 2nd edition. New York: W.W. Norton & Company; 1963.

Printed and bound by CPI Group (UK) Ltd, Croydon, CR0 4YY

03/10/2024

01040479-0004